Edgar L. Patch, Massachusetts College of Pharmacy

Syllabus Of Pharmacy Course

Edgar L. Patch, Massachusetts College of Pharmacy

Syllabus Of Pharmacy Course

ISBN/EAN: 9783741134340

Manufactured in Europe, USA, Canada, Australia, Japa

Cover: Foto ©Lupo / pixelio.de

Manufactured and distributed by brebook publishing software
(www.brebook.com)

Edgar L. Patch, Massachusetts College of Pharmacy

Syllabus Of Pharmacy Course

PHARMACY COURSE.

DEPARTMENT OF PHARMACY,

MASSACHUSETTS COLLEGE OF PHARMACY,

BOSTON, MASS.

––––––––––

By EDGAR L. PATCH, *Ph. G.*

Professor Theory and Practice of Pharmacy.

BOSTON:

MILLS, KNIGHT & CO., PRINTERS, 115 CONGRESS STREET.

1883.

INTRODUCTION.

To better enable the students in the Department of Pharmacy to follow the course of instruction there given, I devised a syllabus, modelled in part upon that proposed by the late Prof. Proctor. It was so well received that, at the request of the Board of Trustees, an interleaved edition has been printed, in form much more convenient than previous issues. It has been hurriedly prepared, and undoubtedly can be much improved, hence the provision of blank pages on which additions and corrections can be made. Being but a mere outline of the course of study, or a synopsis of the lectures, it cannot take the place of the lectures themselves, but may serve as an aid in taking notes upon the principal topics.

E. L. PATCH.

JUNIOR COURSE.

SECTION ONE.

Pharmacy defined. Outline history of pharmacy. European and American pharmacy contrasted. Pharmacy laws. History of the pharmacopœa. Review of last pharmacopœa. Description of dispensatories.

BOOKS OF REFERENCE.

U. S. Pharmacopœa 1880; Parrish's Pharmacy; Proctor's Pharmacy (Bernard Proctor, Eng.); Attfield's Pharm. Chemistry; Lloyd's Chemistry of Medicines; Pareira's Physician's Prescription Book; Mann's Prescription Writing; Rice's Posological Table; Griffith's Formulary; Stewart's Pocket Therapeutics and Dose Book; Dick's Encyclopedia; Gerrish's Prescription Writing; Aids to Chemistry; Semple, 3 Parts.

PHARMACEUTICAL PERIODICALS.

Am. Jour. Pharmacy; New Remedies; Druggist's Circular; Chemist and Druggist; Weekly Drug News; Pharmaceutical Record; The Pharmacist, etc.

SECTION TWO.

Definition and consideration of weight. The balance; principles involved in its construction. How to care for the balance and how to use it. History of derivation of standards of weights and measures, English and Metric.

U. S. STANDARDS.

Standard Yard.—A bronze bar thirty-eight inches long, with plugs of gold sunk an inch from each end, on which the terminal lines of the yard are engraved. Referable to the *length* of a pendulum (39.139 inches), vibrating seconds, in latitude of London, in a vacuum, barometric pressure 30 inches, temperature 62° F.

Standard of Troy and Apoth. Weight.—A brass weight, = 5,760 grains = Troy pound.

Standard of Avcirdupois Weight.—A brass weight, = 7,000 grs. = av. pound.

Standard of Wine Measure.—A gallon, = 231 cu. in. = 58.328 + grs. of water at 62° F., 30 in. barom.

Standard of Dry Measure.—A bushel, = 2,150 + cu. in. 77.6274 av. lbs. water at 62° F., 30 in. barom.

METRIC SYSTEM.

Metre (from Gr. Metron—measure) (Eng. meter) = $\frac{1}{10000000}$ of quadrant, = 39.370 inches.

Sub-divisions	Meter—Mille, from Latin Mille = $\frac{1}{1000}$.			Abbreviated m. m.		
	"	Centi,	"	"	Centum = $\frac{1}{100}$.	"	c. m.
	"	Deci,	"	"	Decem = $\frac{1}{10}$.	"	d. m.
Multiples . .	"	Deka,	"	Greek Deka = 10.		"	D. m.
	"	Hekto,	"	"	Hecaton = 100.	"	H. m.
	"	Kilo,	"	"	Chilioi = 1,000.	"	K. m.
	"	Myria,	"	"	Myrioi = 10,000.	"	M. m

PRONUNCIATION.

Centi in French = Santí (an. as in want) Eng. sĕntĭ.
Chilioi = Kĕ lē oy — hence kīlo, not kĭlo.

ACCENT.

On first syllables. As mil'le méter, ki'lo méter.

Standard of Measure of Weight.—Gramme or gram (from Gr. gramma, a small weight) = weight of cu. c. m. of water at 39° F. or 4° C. = 15.432 grains.

Standard of Measure of Capacity.—Liter (from Gr. litra, a pound) = cu. d. m. = 1000 c. c. = 61.028 cu. in. = 2.113 wine pints.

Standard of Measure of Solidity.—Ster (from Gr. stereos, solid) = 1 cu. m. = 1,000 K. g. = 2,204.6 av. lbs.

Standard of Surface Measure.—Ar (from Latin area, surface) = sq. D. m. = 100 sq. m. = 119.6 sq. yds.

1 gram = 15.432 grs. 1 grain = 0.065 gms. 1 oz. av. = 28.35 gms. 1 troy oz. = 31.103 gms. 1 c. c. = 16.231 minims. 1 minim = 0.062 c. c. 1 fl. oz. = 29.573 c. c.

Conversion of quantities in each system to their equivalent in the other.

Various methods of ascertaining sp. gr. of liquids; implements employed; sp. gr. bottles; hydrometers of different kinds; densimeters. Methods of ascertaining sp. gr. of solids soluble and insoluble in water; of solids lighter and heavier than water. Sp. gr. of gases.

SECTION THREE.

HEAT.

General uses of heat in pharmacy. Definition of and theories regarding heat. Sources of heat; sun, etc., and combustion of solids, liquids and gases in the great variety of furnaces, stoves, lamps and burners,—illustrated by diagrams, models and apparatus. Heating by conduction, convexion and radiation. By reflection. Effects of heat. Structure and use of thermometers. Different kinds of thermometers. Equalization. Application of heat to drying. Steam, hot air and water ovens and drying closets. Desiccators. Drying drugs, gases and utensils.

Drug grinding and powdering by means of mills of various kinds and the pestle and mortar. Cleansing of mills and mortars. Drug sifting. Sieves of silk, hair cloth, iron or brass wire, etc. Considerations governing fineness of powders. Character of commercial powders; Powdering chemicals.

Boiling. Modification of boiling point by pressure of air or vapor,—by nature of containing vessel.

Evaporation. Spontaneous evaporation. Rapidity of evaporation; dependent upon degree of heat; amount of surface exposed to air; upon dryness of air brought in contact with the surface and its freedom of supply. Evaporation in retorts, flasks, capsules. Evaporation of solutions of salts; of solutions of gases; of liquids containing precipitates; of galenical solutions. Evaporation with exclusion of air. Evaporation in vacuo. Estimation of residue.

Heat for evaporation, etc. Sand-bath, water-bath, steam-bath, oil-bath, saturated solutions of salts.

Distillation and its uses. Simple, fractional and destructive distillation. The structure and method of employing the various forms of distillatory apparatus applicable to the chemical and pharmaceutical processes of the pharmacopœa. How to care for and cleanse such apparatus. Sublimation and calcination applied to pharmacopœal uses.

Deliquescence and efflorescence.

EFFECTS OF EXPOSURE TO AIR UPON PHARMACOPŒAL CHEMICALS.

These in this column exposed to moist air absorb moisture and liquify or deliquesce.

These in this column exposed to dry air lose water of crystallization or effloresce.

Acidum Carbolicum.
" Chromicum.
Ammonii Iodidum (badly).
" Nitras.
" Valerianas.
Auri et Sodii Chloridum.
Calcii Bromidum (badly).
" Chloridum "
Ferri " "
Ferri et Ammonii Citras (slightly).
" " Tartras "
" Quininæ Citras "
" Strychninæ " "
Hyoscyaminæ Sulphas.
Lithii Bromidum (badly).
" Citras.
" Salicylas.
Magnesii Citras Granulatus.
Pilocarpinæ Hydrochloras.
Potassa (Potassii Hydras).
" cum Calce.
Potassii Acetas (badly).
" Carbonas (Salt of Tartar).
" Citras.
" Cyanidum.
" Hypophosphis (badly).
" Iodidum (slightly).
" Sulphis "
" Tartras "
Soda (Sodii Hydras).
Sodii Hypophosphis.
" Iodidum.
" Nitras (slightly).
Zinci Bromidum (badly).
" Chloridum "
" Iodidum.

Acidum Citricum.
Codeina.
Cupri Acetas.
" Sulphas (Blue Vitriol).
Ferri et Ammonii Sulphas (Ferric Alum).
Ferri Sulphas (Green Vitriol).
Magnesii Sulphas (Epsom Salts).
Mangani "
Plumbi Acetas (Sugar of Lead).
Potassii et Sodii Tartras (slightly) (Rochelle Salts).
Potassii Ferrocyanidum (Yellow Prussiate of Potassium).
Quininæ Bisulphas.
Soda (Sodii Hydras).
Sodii Acetas.
" Arsenias (slightly).
" Benzoas.
" Boras (Borax).
" Hyposulphis.
" Carbonas (badly).
" Phosphas "
" Sulphas (Glauber's Salt) (badly).
" Sulphis (badly).
Strychninæ Sulphas.
Zinci Acetas.
" Sulphas (White Vitriol).

Ammonii Carbonas—loses CO_2 and NH_3 and becomes bicarbonate

pumps. Hot filtration. Jacketed funnels, steam coils, etc. Continuous filtration. Decolorization. Laws controlling precipitation. Separation, washing, drying and weighing of precipitates. Decantation.

CRYRSTALLIZATION.

Laws governing crystallization. Formation, separation and drying of crystals.

FORM, SOLUBILITY, ETC., OF *SOLUBLE* OFF. CHEMICALS

Common Name.	Officinal.	Form. Figures refer to System of cryst.	Solubility. Parts by weight solving one part of salt.	
			Water 60° F.	Boiling Water.
White Arsenic.	Acidum Arseniosum.	Octahedral. 1	38–80	15
Benzoic Acid.	" Benzoicum.	Feath. needles and plates.	500	15
Boric " Boracic Acid.	" Boricum.	Triclinic. 5 Six-sided plates.	25	3
Carbolic Acid. Phenol.	" Carbolicum.	Trimetric. 3 Needle shaped.	20	
Chromic Acid.	" Chromicum.	Hexagonal. 6 (Crimson needles or columns.)	Freely.	Freely.
Citric "	" Citricum.	Rt.Rhom.Prisms. [5	$\frac{4}{5}$	$\frac{1}{2}$
Gallic "	Gallicum.	Triclinic. 5 Needles or prisms.	100	3
Salicylic.	" Salicylicum.	Monoclinic. 4 Prismatic needles.	450	14
Tartaric Acid.	" Tartaricum.	Monoclinic. 4	$\frac{7}{10}$	$\frac{1}{2}$
Tannic "	" Tannicum.	Light yel. scales. 6	Very.	
Alum.	Alumen.			
Al. et Pot. Sulph.		Octahedral. 1	$10\frac{1}{4}$	$\frac{3}{10}$
Sulphate of Aluminium.	Aluminii Sulphas.	Cryst. powder.	$1\frac{2}{10}$	Very.
Benzoate of Ammonium.	Ammonii Benzoas.	Four-sided laminæ. 5	$1\frac{2}{10}$	
Bromide "	" Bromidum.	Cubical prisms. 1	$1\frac{1}{2}$	$\frac{7}{10}$
Carbonate "	" Carbonas.	Translucent masses.	4	Decomposes.
Chloride "	" Chloridum.	Monometric. 1	3	$1\frac{37}{100}$
Iodide "	" Iodidum.	Cubical. 1	1	$\frac{1}{2}$
Nitrate "	" Nitras.	Rhombic prisms.3	$\frac{1}{2}$	Very.
Phosphate "	" Phosphas.	Monoclinic " 4	4	$\frac{1}{2}$
Sulphate "	" Sulphas.	Rhombic " 3	$1\frac{3}{10}$	1
Valerianate "	" Valerianas.	Quadrangular Plates.	Very.	Very.

12

Common Name.	Officinal.	Form.	Figures refer to System of cryst.	Water 50° F.	Boiling Water.
Tartar Emetic.	Antimonii et Potassii Tartras.	Rhombs.	3	17	3
Hydrochlorate of Apomorphine.	Apomorphinæ Hydrochloras.			$6\frac{8}{10}$	Decomposes.
Nitrate of Silver. Lunar Caustic. Lapis Infernalis.	Argenti Nitras.	Rhombic.	3	$\frac{8}{10}$	$\frac{1}{10}$
Iodide of Arsenic.	Arsenii Iodidum.	Orange red cryt. scales.		$3\frac{1}{2}$	Decomposes.
Atropine.	Atropina.	Prisms.		600	35
Sulphate of Atropine.	Atropinæ Sulphas.	"		$\frac{4}{10}$	Very.
Chloride of Gold and Sodium.	Auri et Sodii Chloridum.	Orange yellow powder.		Very.	Very.
Citrate of Bismuth and Ammonium.	Bismuthi et Ammonii Citras.	Pearly scales.		"	"
Caffeine.	Caffeina.	Silky needles.		75	$9\frac{1}{4}$
Bromide of Calcium.	Calcii Bromidum.	Granular.		$\frac{4}{10}$	Very.
Chloride "	" Chloridum.	{ Off. fused. Hexagonal.	6	$1\frac{1}{2}$	"
Hypophosphite "	" Hypophosphis.	Six-sided prisms.	6	$6\frac{4}{10}$	6
Chloral. Hydrate of Chloral.	Chloral.	Rhomboidal.	6	Very.	Very.
Sulphate of Cinchonidine.	Cinchonidinæ Sulphas.	White needles or prisms.		100	4
Cinchonine.	Cinchonina.	White needles or prisms.		Little.	Little.
Sulphate of Cinchonine.	Cinchoninæ Sulphas.	Prisms.		70	14
Codeine.	Codeina.	Rhombic prisms.	3	80	17
Acetate of Copper.	Cupri Acetas.	Bluish green prisms.		15	5
Sulphate " Blue Vitriol. Blue Stone.	" Sulphas.	*Blue* triclinic.	5	$2\frac{4}{10}$	$\frac{1}{4}$
Chloride of Iron.	Ferri Chloridum.	Orange yellow cryst. masses.		Very.	Very.
Ferric Alum. Ammonio-ferric Alum. " " Sulphate.	Ferri et Ammonii Sulphas.	Octahedral. (Pale violet.)	1	3	$\frac{8}{10}$
Lactate of Iron.	Ferri Lactas.	Greenish white cryst. crusts.		40	12
Sulphate " Green Vitriol. Copperas.	Ferri Sulphas.	Monoclinic. (Green.)	4	$1\frac{4}{10}$	$\frac{3}{10}$

Parts by weight solving one part of salt.

Common Name.	Officinal.	Form. Figures refer to System of cryst.	Solubility. Parts by weight solving one part of salt. Water 59° F.	Boiling Water.
Corrosive Sublimate. Mercuric Chloride. Oxymuriate Merc. Oxychloride " Bichloride " Perchloride "	Hydrargyri Chloridum. Corrosivum.	Rhombic prisms. [3	16	2
Cyanide of Mercury.	HydrargyriCyanidum.	Prisms (Quadratic). 2	$12\frac{8}{16}$	3
Sulphate of Hyoscyamine.	Hyoscyaminæ Sulphas.	Yellowish scales.	Very.	Very.
Benzoate of Lithium.	Lithii Benzoas.	Powdery scales.	4	$2\frac{1}{2}$
Bromide "	" Bromidum.	Granular.	Very.	Very.
Citrate "	" Citras.	Powder.	$5\frac{1}{2}$	$2\frac{1}{4}$
Salicylate "	" Salicylas.	"	Very.	Very.
Epsom Salts.	Magnesii Sulphas.	Rt. Rhombic prisms. 3	$\frac{8}{16}$	$\frac{1}{4}$
Sulphite of Magnesium.	" Sulphis.	Cryst. powder.	20	19
Sulphate of Manganese.	Mangani Sulphas.	Rt. Rhombic prisms. 3 (Rose color.)	$\frac{8}{16}$	$\frac{8}{16}$
Morphine.	Morphina.	Prismatic. 3		500
Acetate of Morph.	Morphinæ Acetas.	Powder.	12	$1\frac{1}{2}$
Hydrochlorate of Morph.	" Hydrochloras.	Feathery cryst.	24	$\frac{1}{4}$
Sulphate of "	" Sulphas.	" "	24	$\frac{1}{4}$
Salicylate of Physostigmine.	Pysostigminæ Salicylas.	White or reddish columnar cryst.	130	30
Picrotoxin.	Picrotoxinum.	Prismatic. 3	150	25
Hydrochlorate of Pilocarpine.	Pilocarpinæ Hydrochloras.		Very.	Very.
Acetate of Lead. Sugar " Sal. Saturni.	Plumbi Acetas.	Monoclinic prisms. 4	$1\frac{8}{16}$	$\frac{1}{2}$
Nitrate of Lead.	" Nitras.	Octahedral.	2	$\frac{8}{16}$
Caustic Potash.	Potassa.	Pencils.	$\frac{1}{2}$	Very.
Acetate of Potassium.	Potassii Acetas.	Granular powder.	$\frac{8}{16}$	Very.
Bicarbonate "	" Bicarbonas.	Monoclinic. 4 Four-sided prisms.	$3\frac{1}{2}$	Decomposes.
Bichromate "	" Bichromas.	Triclinic. 5 (Orange red.)	10	$1\frac{1}{2}$
Bitartrate " Cream of Tartar.	" Bitartras.	Rhombic cryst. 3	210	15
Bromide of Potassium.	" Bromidum.	Cubical. 1	$1\frac{8}{16}$	1
Carbonate "	" Carbonas.	Gran. powd. 1	$\frac{8}{16}$	$\frac{1}{10}$

Common Name.	Officinal.	Form. Figures refer to System of cryst.	Solubility. Parts by weight solving one part of salt. Water 59° F.	Boiling Water
Chlorate Potassium.	Potassii. Chloras.	Monoclinic plates. 4	16¼	2
Citrate "	" Citras.	Gran. powd.	$\frac{6}{10}$	Very
Cyanide "	" Cyanidum.	" " or amorph. masses.	2	1
Rochelle Salts.	Potassii et Sodii Tartras.	Rhombic. 3	2½	Very.
Yellow Prussiate of Potassium.	Potassii Ferrocyanidum.	Four-sided prisms. 2	4	2
Hypophosphite of Potassium.	Potassii Hypophosphis.	Hexagonal or Gran. powder. 6	$\frac{6}{10}$	$\frac{3}{10}$
Iodide of Potassium.	Potassii Iodidum.	Cubical. 1	$\frac{6}{10}$	$\frac{5}{10}$
Nitrate " Saltpetre. Nitre.	" Nitras.	Rhombic. 3 Six-sided prisms.	4	$\frac{4}{10}$
Permanganate of Potassium.	" Permanganas.	Purple Rhom. prisms. Needle shape. 3	20	3
Sulphate of Potassium.	" Sulphas.	Rhombic prisms.3	9	4
Sulphite "	" Sulphis.	Rhombic Octahedral. 4	4	5
Tartrate "	" Tartras.	Monoclinic. 4	$\frac{7}{10}$	$\frac{5}{10}$
Sulphate of Quinidine.	Quinidinæ Sulphas.	Silky needles.	100	7
Quinine.	Quinina.	Flaky powder.	1000	700
Bisulphate of Quinine.	Quininæ Bisulphas.	Needle shape.	10	Very.
Hydrobromate "	" Hydrobromas.	" "	16	1
Hydrochlorate "	" Hydrochloras.	" "	34	1
Sulphate "	" Sulphas.	" "	740	30
Valerianate "	" Valerianas.	Triclinic. 5	100	40
Sugar.	Saccharum.	Monoclinic. 4	$\frac{5}{10}$	$\frac{2}{10}$
Sugar of Milk.	Saccharum Lactis.	Trimetric. 3	7	1
Salicin.	Salicinum.	Tabular.	28	$\frac{7}{10}$
Santonin.	Santoninum.	Prismatic.		250
Caustic Soda.	Soda.	Opaque masses.	$1\frac{7}{10}$	$\frac{7}{10}$
Acetate of Sodium.	Sodii Acetas.	Monoclinic prisms. 4	3	1
Arseniate "	" Arsenias.	Prismatic oblique. [4	4	Very.
Benzoate "	" Benzoas.	Powder.	$1\frac{6}{10}$	$1\frac{3}{10}$
Bicarbonate "	" Bicarbonas.	Powder. 4 Pure=Monoclinic	12	Decomposes.
Bisulphite "	" Bisulphis.	Prismatic.	4	2

Common Name.	Officinal.	Form.		Solubility.	
		Figures refer to System of cryst.		Parts by weight solving one part of salt.	
				Water 35°F.	Boiling Water.
Borax.	Sodii Boras.	Monoclinic.	4	16	$\frac{1}{2}$
Bromide of Sodium.	" Bromidum.	"		$1\frac{1}{2}$	$\frac{7}{10}$
Carbonate " Sal Soda.	" Carbonas.	"	4	$1\frac{6}{10}$	$\frac{1}{4}$
Chlorate "	" Chloras.	Reg. Tetrahedrons.	1	$1\frac{1}{10}$	$\frac{1}{2}$
Chloride " Common Salt.	" Chloridum.	Cubical.	1	$2\frac{8}{10}$	$2\frac{1}{4}$
Hypophosphite of Sodium.	" Hypophosphis.	Tabular plates.	1		$\frac{1}{10}$
Hyposulphite of Sodium.	" Hyposulphis.	Monoclinic prisms.	4	$1\frac{1}{2}$	$\frac{1}{4}$
Iodide of Sodium.	" Iodidum.	" "	4	$\frac{6}{10}$	$\frac{3}{10}$
Nitrate "	" Nitras.	Rhombohedral.	6	$1\frac{3}{10}$	$1\frac{5}{10}$
Phosphate "	" Phosphas.	Monoclinic.	4	6	2
Pyrophosphate "	" Pyrophosphas.	"	4	12	$1\frac{1}{10}$
Salicylate "	" Salicylas.	Quadrangular prisms.	2	$1\frac{1}{2}$	Very.
Santoninate "	" Santoninas.	Rhombic.	3	3	$\frac{1}{4}$
Sulphate " Glauber's salt.	" Sulphas.	Monoclinic.	4	$2\frac{8}{10}$	$\frac{1}{4}$
Sulphite of Sodium.	" Sulphis.	"	4	4	$\frac{9}{10}$
Sulphocarbolate of Sodium.	" Sulphocarbolas.	Rhombic prisms.			
Strychnine.	Strychnina.	Octahedral.	1	6700	2500
Sulphate of Strychnine.	Strychninæ Sulphas.	Prisms.		10	2
Thymol.	Thymol.	Hexagonal.	6	1200	900
Acetate of Zinc.	Zinci Acetas.	Six-sided tables.	3		$1\frac{1}{2}$
Bromide "	" Bromidum.	Gran. powd.		Very.	Very.
Chloride "	" Chloridum.	" "		"	"
Iodide "	" Iodidum.	Octahedral or gran. powd.	1		
Sulphate " White Vitriol.	" Sulphas.	Right rhomb prisms.	3	$1\frac{6}{10}$	$1\frac{3}{10}$
Valerianate of Zinc.	" Valerianas.	Pearly scales.		100	Decomposes.

SECTION FIVE.

NOMENCLATURE OF CHEMICALS.

Definition of Terms. — Salts, bases, acids, oxides, hydroxides, hydrates, hydrides, anhydrides.

Definition of Prefixes.—Meta, pyro, hyper, per, hypo, proto, bin, deuto, sesqui, ter, tri, super, sub.
Definition of Terminations.—Application.

SECTION SIX.

Maceration and Digestion; their theory and practice.

PERCOLATION.

Brief history and latest theories. Principles involved. Forms of percolators. Preparing the drug. Moistening and packing. Rate of flow. The percolate. Continuous percolation. Repercolation.

SECTION SEVEN.

The Classes of Preparations, defined and described. — Aquæ, Liquores, Infusa, Decocta, Mucilagines, Syrupi, Spiritus, Tincturæ, Vina, Extracta Fluida, Aceta, Oleoresinæ, Glycerita, Mellita, Oxymellita, Misturæ, Confectiones, Extracta, Abstracta, Trochisci, Pulveres, Pilulæ, Chartæ, Cerata, Unguenta, Suppositoria, Oleata, Linimenta, Emplastra.

SECTION EIGHT.

DISPENSING PHARMACY.

Care of stock. Concentrated solutions for dispensing. Weighing and measuring. Mortars. Pestles. Spatulas of steel, silver, horn, ivory and glass. Ointment and pill tiles. Other apparatus. The cleansing of apparatus and utensils.
The Prescription Counter. Its management and furnishing.

THE PRESCRIPTION.

Its reading and interpretation. Copying. Labelling. Typical prescriptions, demonstrating peculiarities of chirography, abbreviations, incompatibles, omissions, overdoses, etc.

MIXTURES.

Chemically incompatible. Therapeutically incompatible. Altered by exposure to heat, air or light. Emulsions of volatile and fixed oils. Difficult examples.

POWDERS.

Mixing of powders that vary in density in small and large masses. Dividing by measure and weight. Deliquescent, efflorescent and volatile powders. Cachets; wafers; capsules.

PILLS.

How to form SOLUBLE, *adhesive*, plastic masses. Combining volatile oils with pill masses. How divide. How finish. Coating with paraffin, tolu, sandarac, sugar, gelatin, etc. Difficult and peculiar masses.

SUPPOSITORIES.

Hot and cold processes. Home made and other moulds. Ointments. Troches. Plasters.

SENIOR COURSE.

THE PREPARATIONS OF THE PHARMACOPŒIA.

Their Source, Manufacture and Employment.

CELLULIN.

Used in natural conditions as filtering media and as surgical dressing.

Common Name.	Botanical Name.	Geog. Source.
Cotton fibre.	Gossypium herbaceum, etc.	(Off.) Semi-tropics.
Flax or linen.	Linum usitatissimum.	Temp. climes.
Hemp.	Cannabis sativa.	E. I. and tem. lat.
Tow.	Short fibre of flax or hemp.	
Oakum.	Old hemp rope, shredded.	
Jute.	Varieties of corchorus.	E. I. and So. U. S.
Manilla.	Musa textilis. (Same genus as banana.)	Phil. Islands.
Ramie, China Grass.	Bœhmeria nivea.	E. I.

ACTION OF STRONG ACIDS ON CELLULIN.

$H_2 SO_4$—cold—dissolves it and forms dextrine.
  do.   —hot —chars it.
$H NO_3$—90° F—forms Gun-cotton, in which nitrile replaces a portion of H in cellulin.

(Higher nitrogenized cotten used in gunnery; the lower known as pyróxylin (off.) Pyroxylinum, used in collodions,—Collodium, Collodium Flexile, Collodium cum Cantharide, Collodium Stypticum.)

$H Cl$.—boiled—dissolves it as cellulin.

ACTION OF DILUTE ACIDS.

$H_2 SO_4$—boiled=dextrin and glucose.
$H NO_3$ — do.   (Sp. gr. 1, 2)=Oxalic Acid.

ACTION OF STRONG ALKALIES.

Na HO. or K HO. dissolve very slightly and change to starch and gum.
 do.   do.   —heated—form Oxalic Acid.
       (Weaker alkalies form paper pulp).

DESTRUCTIVE DISTILLATION.

Residue = charcoal—off.—Carbo Ligni.

Distillate = 1. Tarry bodies, resins, creasote, etc. 2. Aqueous solution pyroligneous acid, methylic alcohol, acetone, etc.

No. 2 + Ca 2 HO fixes $H\bar{A}$ as Ca $\bar{A}_2$. Distill mixture and residual solution of Ca $\bar{A}_2$ + Na_2 SO_4 = Ca SO_4 + 2 Na $\bar{A}$. From Na $\bar{A}$ purified by heat, solution and crytallization + H_2 SO_4 comes

Acidum Aceticum—off. Ext. Colch. Rad. (used in all acetates,—very unstable salts).

Acidum Aceticum Dilutum.—Off. Aceta, Emp. Ammoniaci, Liq. Am. Acet., Syr. Allii, Syr. Scillæ.

From anhydrous Na $\bar{A}$ + H_2 SO_4 comes Acidum Aceticum Glaciale (off.).

Distillate from No. 2 mixture contains methylic alcohol and acetone.

Add Ca Cl_2 and distill acetone.

Add residue (= Ca Cl_2 + CH_3 HO), to water, and distill methylic alcohol.

STARCHES.

The following list comprises those bodies whose virtue depends in whole or in part upon starch:

Common Name.	Officinal Name.	Bot. Source.	Geog. Source.
Acorns.		Genus Quercus.	Temp. Lat.
Arrowroot.		Maranta-aurandinacea.	E. and W. I.
Barley, 66%.		Hordeum distichon.	Temp. Lat.
Beans, 33%.		Faba vulgaris. Phaseolus "	do.
Chestnuts and other edible nuts.		Castanea vesca, etc.	do.
Corn, 67%.		Zea Mays.	do.
Oats, 60%. Divested of husks form groats.		Avena Sativa.	do.
Peas, 37%.		Pisum sativum.	do.
Potatoes, 20%.		Solanum Tuberosa.	America.
Sweet Potatoes, 16%.		Convolvulus batatus.	Am. or E. I. (?)

Common Name.	*Officinal Name.*	*Bot. Source.*	*Geog. Source.*
Rye, 64%.		Secale cereale.	Temp. Lat.
Rice, 88%.		Oryza sativa.	(?)
Sago.		Metroxylon Sagus.	
		Sagus Reumphü.	E. I.
Tapioca. ⎫ Cassava. ⎬ Manioc. ⎭		Janipha Manihot.	S. A.
Wheat, 57%.	⎧ Amylum. ⎨ Amylum Iodatum. ⎩ Glyceritum Amyli.	Triticum vulgare.	Temp. Lat

BODIES THAT CONTAIN STARCH IN NOTABLE QUANTITY.

Common Name.	*Officinal Name.*	*Bot. Source.*	*Geog. Source.*
Cacao Seeds.		Theobroma Cacao.	Brazil and Trop. Am.
Canary Seeds. ⎫ Phalaris. ⎬		Phalaris canariensis.	Basin of Mediter· ranean Sea.
Hemidesmus. ⎫ Indian Sarsap. ⎬		Hemidesmus indicus.	India.
Orris Root.		Iris Florentina.	So. Eu.
Wild Yam Root.		Dioscorea villosa.	U. S.

BODIES THAT CONTAIN INULIN IN NOTABLE QUANTITY.

Common Name.	*Officinal Name.*	*Bot. Source.*	*Geog. Source.*
Arnica Root.		Arnica montana.	Eu.
Artichoke Root, Jer.		Helianthus tuberosus.	Eu.
Burdock "	Lappa.	Lappa officinalis.	Eu. and N. A.
Chicory "		Cichorium intybus.	Eu., U. S.
Colchicum "	Colchici Radix. Ext., Fl. Ext.,Vin.	Colchicum autumnale.	Eu.
Dahlia "		Dahlia variabilis.	Mexico.
Dandelion "	Taraxacum. Ext. and Fl. Ext.	Taraxacum Dens Leonis.	U. S.
Elecampane "	Inula.	Inula helenium.	No. Eu.

BODIES ALLIED TO STARCHES IN THEIR USES.

Common Name.	*Officinal Name.*	*Bot. Source.*	*Geog. Source.*
Salep.		Orchis mascula.	Eu. and As.
Irish Moss. ⎫ Carrageen. ⎬	Chondrus.	Chondrus crispus.	W. Eu. and N. A.
Iceland Moss.	Cetraria Off. in Dec. Cetraria.	Cetraria islandica.	Iceland, etc.

MUCILAGINOUS DRUGS

Containing soluble gum known as *Arabin*, said to be a bigummate of calcium, Soluble gum known as Dextrine, Insoluble gum known as Bassorin, and modifications of same. Gums are employed as demulcents, as vehicles for the suspension of insoluble solids in mixtures, and to separate fatty particles in emulsions.

REACTIONS OF ARABIN.

Soluble in its own weight of water. Insoluble in Alcohol, Ether and Oils. Ppt. from solution by Sol. Subacet. Lead, Potassic Silicate, Alcohol, Ether. Gelatinized by Ferric Chloride and Borax.

ACTION OF ACIDS.

Strong H_2SO_4, with heat, chars it.

Dilute H_2SO_4, with heat = non-fermentable glucose = arabinose.

Strong HNO_3, converts into mucic acid, with traces of oxalic, tartaric and saccharic acids.

ACTION OF ALKALIES.

Alkalies and alkaline earths form soluble compounds.

REACTIONS OF BASSORIN.

Swells in water, hot or cold. Insoluble in Alcohol, Ether and Oils. Soluble in HNO_3 Dil., in H Cl Dil., and in Liq. Ammon. Strong HNO_3 converts into mucic and oxalic acids.

Arabic acid = $C_{12}H_{22}O_{11}$. Dextrin and Bassorin $C_6H_{10}O_5$.

TABLE 1, CONTAINING ARABIN OR MODIFICATIONS.

Common Name.	Officinal Name.	Botanical Source.	Geog. Source.
Gum Arabic.	{ Acacia. { Mucil. and Syr.	Acacia vera, etc.	Asia, Africa, etc.
Blue-weed.		Echium vulgare.	Europe.
Borage-root.		Borago officinale.	Levant.
Hound's Tongue.		Cynoglossum officinale.	Europe and U. S.
Lungwort.		Pulmonaria officinalis.	Europe.
Marshmallow Root and flowers.	Althœa. Syrup. (root).	Althea officinale.	Asia Minor & Eu.
Mezquite gum.		Algarobia glandulosa.	Texas, N.Mex.etc.
Okra, or Gombo capsules.		Hibiscus esculentus.	Africa.
Virginia Lungwort.		Pulmonaria Virginica.	United States.

TABLE 2, CONTAINING BASSORIN OR MODIFICATIONS.

Common Name.	Officinal Name.	Botanical Source.	Geog. Source.
Bael fruit.		Ægle marmalos.	India.
Baobab.		Adansonia digitata.	Trop. Africa.
Bassora, or Kutera-gum.		Unknown.	Persia & Greece.
Benne leaves.		Sesamum Indicum.	India.
Bashew nut.		Anacardium occidentale.	Trop. America.
Comfrey root.		Symphytum officinale.	Europe.
Evening Primrose.		Œnothera biennis.	North America.
Flaxseed.	Linum.	Linum usitatissimum.	So. Europe.
Hog, or Doctor gum.		Rhus metopium.	So. America.
Jujube berries.		Zizyphus vulgaris.	Originally Asia Minor & Greece.
Quince seeds.	Cyndonium(Muc).	Cydonia vulgaris.	Ditto.
Sassafras pith.	Sassafras medulla (Muc).	Sassafras officinale.	No. America.
Slippery Elm.	Ulmus (Muc).	Ulmus fulva.	United States.
Tragacanth.	Tragacantha (Muc).	Astragalus verus.	Asia Minor and Persia.

Gums are infusible, non-volatile, amorphous bodies, destitute of N., distinguished from resins by their softening in water and insolubility in alcohol; from starches by their softening in cold water; from sugars by being non-fermentable from simple exposure, and with HNO_3 forming mucic acid.

STARCH AND SUGAR.

STARCH.

Sp. gr. about 1. 5. Insoluble in cold water, alcohol or ether. Soluble in hot water. Employed as a nutrient.

ACTION OF HEAT.

Dry heat 320—350° F. = dextrine. Higher heat = C., CO_2., HĀ. etc.

ACTION OF REAGENTS.

Ppt: from solution by Ca 2HO, Ba 2HO, tannin, alcohol and Sol. Subacet. Lead.

Strong HNO_3 = Xyloidin $C_{18} H_{27} (NO_2)_5 O_{15}$.
Weaker " = Oxalic acid. Still weaker = dextrin.
H Cl., $H_2 C_2 O_4$, H_2 Tä, convert to glucose.
Strong $H_2 SO_4$, dissolves, forming compound acid.
Dilute $H_2 SO_4$ + heat = glucose (amylose).
Dry, strong alkalies + heat = oxalic acid.
Soluble in solutions of alkalies.
Turned blue by Iodine. Grain, moistened, allowed to germinate, dried = malt. (Off. Maltum. Extractum Malti.) With diastase (malt) starch changes to maltose (modification of glucose, $C_{12} H_{22} O_{11} H_2O = 2C_6 H_{12} O_6$).
Starch with malt and yeast, fermented, distilled, = whiskey (off. Spts. Frumenti).
Malt with hops and yeast = beer (lager, ale, porter).

SUB-VARIETIES OF STARCH.

Inulin.—Becomes dextrin by long boiling with water. With iodine no action (or brown color). With dilute acids = lævulose.

Paramylon, glycogen or animal starch, found in lower animals, and in certain viscera of the higher animals. + acids = glucose. + I. no action.

SUGARS.

(a) Saccharoses = $C_{12} H_{22} O_{11}$. (b) Glucoses = $C_6 H_{12} O_6$.
a 1. Cane Sugar. Saccharum (Off). Sugar cane, beets, maple, etc.
2. Milk Sugar (Lactose). Sac. Lactis (Off). From Milk-whey.
3. Melitose from Eucalyptus.
4. Melizitose — Larch.
5. Trehalose — Syrian Manna.
6. Mycose — Ergot.

SOLUBILITIES AND REACTIONS OF CANE SUGAR. (a)

Sp. gr. 1-6. Sol. ½ weight of water, cold:—more in hot. Insol. in alcohol, ether and chloroform.
Strong $H_2 SO_4$ — *chars*. HNO_3 = oxalic and saccharic acids.
Strong H Cl =ulmin and ulmic acids. Dilute mineral and vegetable acids + heat, change from unfermentable sugar to fermentable dextrose and lacvulose.
Weak alkalies little action. Stronger = sucrates. Dry, is not colored brown by dry alkalies.
Reduces alkaline solution of copper — slowly.
Triturated + $KClO_3$ = explosive. + Pb. O_2 takes fire.

ACTION OF HEAT.

360–365° F. melts; cooled = invert sugar. Moistened, melted and cooled = *barley candy.*

400–420° F. parts with H_2O and becomes *caramel.*

Higher heat decomposes = inflammable gases, acetone, aldehyde, $H\bar{A}$., carbon, etc.

Ferments, changes to glucose,—then to alcohol.

Solution invert sugar (molasses, Syr. Fuscus) + yeast, fermented and distilled = rum.

For consideration of glucoses, see "Glucoses and Alcohols."

GLUCOSES AND ALCOHOLS.

Glucose — $C_6 H_{12} O_6$ = Grape Sugar = Dextro-glucose.

1. Found native in sweet fruits, chestnuts, vegetable mould, urine, in liver and stomach during digestion, in honey, etc.

2. Laevulose — In honey, ripe fruit, etc., with glucose.

3. Sorbite — Mountain Ash.

4. Inosite — sugar of muscle.

SOLUBILITIES AND REACTIONS.

Freely soluble in water. Insoluble in alcohol. At 338° F. parts with H_2O and becomes $C_6 H_{10} O_5$ (Glucosan). Higher heat = caramel. H_2SO_4, *does not char.* = Sulpho-saccharic acid. HNO_3 = Oxalic and saccharic acids.

Alkalies — *turn brown.* Reduces alkaline copper solution, *quickly.* Ferments change *at once* to alcohol.

Fruit juices fermented, yield wines. (Off. Vin. Album, Vin. Album Fortius, Vin. Rubrum.)

Wines distilled yield brandies. (Spts. Vini Gallici, off.)

ALCOHOLS.

Hydrocarbons less one or more atoms of H, plus one or more molecules of HO, hence hydroxides of organic bases.

Common Alcohol — from fermentation of sugars. $C_2 H_5 HO$ = Ethyl Hydroxide.

Methylic Alcohol — from dest. dist. of wood, etc. $CH_3 HO$ = Methyl Hydroxide.

Amylic Alcohol — from fermentation of starch sugar, etc. $C_5 H_{11} HO$ = Amyl Hydroxide.

Phenylic Alcohol — from dest. dist. coal, etc. $C_6 H_5 HO$ = Phenyl Hydroxide = Carbolic acid.

Propenylic Alcohol — from fats, etc = glycerine. C_2 H_5 $3HO$ Propenyl Hydroxide.

REACTIONS.

Primary Alcohols $+ O =$ aldehydes.   Aldehydes $+ O =$ acids.   (Ethylic alcohol C_2 H_5 $HO + O = H_2 O + C_2 H_4 O =$ acetic aldehyd. $+ O = C_2 H_4 O_2 =$ acetic acid.)

Amylic Alcohol $+ O =$ amylic aldehyd, $+ O =$ amylic or valerianic acid.

Primary Alcohols form 1.   Oxyethers; — by replacing HO with O, as $(C_2 H_5)_2$ $O = common ether.$

2. *Haloid ethers;* — by replacing HO with halogens, as C_2 H_5 Br. $=$ Hydrobromic Ether.

3. *Compound ethers;* — by replacing HO with compound acid radicals, as C_2 H_5 $NO_2 =$ Nitrous Ether.

4. *Complex ethers;* — by the acid radical replacing the HO from more than one alcohol radical, as CH_3,C_2 H_5 $O =$ methyl, ethyl ether.

ETHYLIC ALCOHOL.

$+ H_2 SO_4 =$ Ether and Etherial oil.   (Hoffman's anodyne.)

$+ HNO_3 =$ Nitrous Ether.   (Sweet Spirits of Nitre.)

$+ Cl.$ and an alkali $(CaHClO_2) =$ Chloroform.

$+ I.$ and an alkali $(K HCO_3) =$ Iodoform.

$+ Br.$ and an alkali $=$ Bromoform.

$+ Cl$ (the alcohol absolute) $=$ Chloral.

AMYLIC ALCOHOL.

$+ HNO_3 =$ Amyl Nitrite. $+ H_2 SO_4 + HNO_3 =$ Amyl Nitrate.   Propenyl Alcohol $+ HNO_3 + H_2 SO_4 =$ Glonoin or Nito glycerin.

TARTRATES, CITRATES AND MALATES.

Tartaric Acid.—$H_2 C_4 H_4 O_6$ or H_2 Tä.

Source—Argols or crude tartar of wines, — impure cream of tartar,— potassic bitartrate, KH Tä.   Purified by dissolving, decolorizing with clay and animal C., concentrating and crystallizing many times, freeing from Ca Tä with H Cl Dil., washing, adding Ca CO_3 + Ca Cl_2 to decompose KH Tä and form Ca Tä, which is washed and decomposed with H_2 SO_4 as— Ca Tä $+ H_2 SO_4 =$ Ca SO_4 + H_2 Tä.

COMPOUNDS OF H_2 Tä.

KH Tä + SbO $=$ K SbO Tä—Anhydrous tartar emetic.   Vin. Ant., Syr. Scillæ Co.

6 KH Tä + Fe$_2$ 6HO = 6 H$_2$ O + K_6 Fe_2 6 $Tä$ (?) Ferri et Potassii Tartras.

2 KH Tä + K$_2$ CO$_3$ = H$_2$ O + CO$_2$ + 2 K_2 $Tä$. Potassii Tartras.

2 KH Tä + Na$_2$ CO$_3$ = H$_2$ O + CO$_2$ + 2 K Na $Tä$, Rochelle Salts, Potassii et Sodii Tartras.

KH Tä 65 parts, Pulv. Jalap. 35 parts = Pulv. Jalapæ Comp.

2 H$_2$ Tä + Am$_2$ CO$_3$ = H$_2$ O + CO$_2$ + 2 Am. H Tä. Ammon Bitart.

4 Am. H Tä + Fe$_2$ 6HO = 4 H$_2$ O + 2 Am. HO + Fe_2 Am_2 4 $Tä$. Ferri et Ammonii Tartras.

H$_2$ Tä (1–7 Gms.) + NaHCO$_3$ (2 Gms.) = Soda Powders. *Not Off.*

H$_2$ Tä (2–25 Gms.) + NaHCO$_3$ (2–58 Gms.) + Nä K Tä (7–75 Gms.) = Seidlitz Powders, Pulv. Effervescens Compositus.

Citric Acid.—H$_3$ C$_6$ H$_5$ O$_7$ or H$_3$ Cï.

Source—Juice of limes, tamarinds, lemons, citrons, etc.   Lemon juice (off.) contains 7–11% H$_3$ Cï. Mist. Potassii Citratis. Syrupus Limonis.

Lime juice—commercial source of H$_3$ Cï.   Clarified by boiling, neutralized + Ca CO$_3$ + Ca (HO)$_2$, boiled, strained hot, the Ca$_3$ 2 Cï washed with hot water and decomposed with H$_2$ SO$_4$.

Ca$_3$ 2 Cï + 3 H$_2$ SO$_4$ = 3 Ca SO$_4$ + 2 H_3 $Cï$—Citric acid.

2 H$_3$ Cï + Fe$_2$ 6 HO = 6 H_2 O, 2 Fe $Cï$ Ferri Citras.   Liquor Ferri Citratis.

Sol. Fe Çï + Am HO = Ferri et Ammonii Citras.

Ferri et Am. Cit. 98 parts, Strychnine 1 part and H$_3$ Cï 1 part = Ferri et Strychninæ Citras.

65 Am. et Fe. Cit., 12 Quinine, 28 H$_3$ Cï, 30 Alc., H$_2$ O q.s. = Liquor Ferri et Quininæ Citratis.

Ferri Cit. 88, Quinine 12, H$_2$ O q. s. = Ferri et Quininæ Citras.

H$_3$ Cï + 3 KH CO$_3$ = K_3 $Cï$ (Potassii Citras). (Liquor Potassii Citratis) + 3 CO$_2$ + 3 H$_2$O.

2 H$_3$ Cï + 3 Li$_2$ CO$_3$ = 3 CO$_2$ + 3 H$_2$ O + 2 Li_3 $Cï$—Lithii Citras,

13 Mag. Carb., 26 H$_3$ Cï, 80 Syr. Acid Cit., 2 KHCO$_3$, H$_2$ O q.s. = Liquor Magnesii Citratis.

11 Mag. Carb., + 48 H$_3$ Cï, + 37 Na HCO$_3$, + 8 No. 60 Sugar, + Alc. q.s. and H$_2$ O q.s. = Magnesii Citras Granulatus.

H$_3$ Cï + Bi ONO$_3$ = HNO$_3$ + H$_2$ O + Bi Ci = Bismuthi Citras.

Bi Ci + Am. HO = Bismuthi et Ammonii Citras.

8 H$_3$ Cï, 8 H$_2$ O, 4 Spts. Limonis, 980 Syr. = Syrupus Acidi Citrici.

Malic Acid.—H$_3$ C$_4$ H$_3$ O$_5$—H$_3$ Mä.

Source—Juice of apples, gooseberries, *rhubarb* stalks, etc.

Pb$_3$ 2 Mä insoluble in Am. HO, Pb$_3$ 2 Cï and Pb Tä soluble.

Ca$_3$ Cï insoluble in KHO, Ca Tä soluble in KHO.

VOLATILE OILS.

Mostly liquids lighter than water, odorous, volatile, distil with water, little soluble in water, soluble in strong alcohol, ether, chloroform, benzole and fixed oils. Carminatives and stimulants. Those marked Aq. are officinal in Aquæ; Sp. in Spiritus; Tr. in Trochisci; Pil. in Pilulæ.

CLASS 1. TERPENES. $C_{10} H_{16}$. BINARY (2 ELEMENTS).

Common Name.	Off. Name.	Botanical Source.	Geog. Source.
Oil of Amber.	Oleum Succini.	Fosil resin,–Amber	So. E. Eu.
" Bergamot.	" Bergamii. Spt.Odoratus	Citrus Bergamia.	do. Italy.
" Bitter Orange. ⎫ Bigarade. ⎪ Seville. ⎬ " Sweet Orange. ⎪ Portugal " ⎭	" Aurantii Corticis. Elix.Au.,Spts. Au.	Citrus Vulgaris, Amara (peel).	So.Eu.,W.I.&c.
	Spts.Myrciæ.	Citrus Aurantium (peel).	do.
" Neroli. Orange Flowers.	" Aurantii Florum. Spts.Odoratus.	Flowers of both named var. O.	do.
" Black Pepper.		Piper nigrum (fruit).	Tropics.
" Copaiba.	" Copaibæ.	By dist.from Copaiba with $H_2 O$.	S. A.
" Cajeput.	" Cajuputi.	Melalenca Cajuputi (leaves).	E. I. $C_{10} H_{16}$ H_2O.
" Cubebs.	" Cubebæ.	Cubeba officinalis (unripe fruit).	E. I.
" Fir.		Abies balsamea.	N. A.
" Galbanum.		Galbanum—gumresin, from Ferula galbaniflua.	No. Persia.
" Hemlock. Spruce.		Abies canadensis (branches).	U. S.
" Juniper.	" Juniperi. Sp.&Co.Sp.	Juniperus communis (berries).	N. A. and Eu.
" Lavender.	" Lavandulæ. Tr.Lav.Co.	Lav. vera. (flowers and plant).	Eng., France.
" Lavender Flowers.	" Lavandulæ Florum. Spts. Lavand. " Odoratus. " Ammon.Aro.	Fresh Lavender.	" "
" Lemon.	" Limonis. Sp. Am. Aro. Spts. Odoratus.	Citrus Limonem.	So. Eu.

Common Name.	Off. Name.	Botanical Source.	Geog. Source.
Oil of Sage.	Oleum	Salvia officinalis.	Eu. and U. S.
" Savin.	" Sabinæ.	Juniperus sabina (branches).	"　　"
" Turpentine,	" Terebinthinæ Lin. Canth. Lin. Tereb.	From Pines.	"　　"

CLASS 2. OXYGENATED. (C_{10} H_{16} OXYDIZED ?) TERNARY.

Common Name.	Off. Name.	Botanical Source.	Geog. Source.
Oil of Anise.	Oleum Anisi. Aq., Sp., Tr.Opii Camph.	Seeds of Pimpi- nella anisum and Illicium anisa- tum.	So. and Cen.Eu., E.Asia.$C_{10}H_{16}$ & anethol $C_{10}H_{12}O$.
" Arbor Vitæ. White Cedar (Thujæ).		Thuja occidentalis (branches).	N. A.
" Bay. Wild Clove. " Cin'amon.	" Myrciæ. Spts.Myrciæ.	Myrcia acris (leaves).	W. I. and Venezuela. Like Oil Cloves.
" Bayberries.		Laurus nobilis.	Lavant.
" Camphor.		Camph.officinarum.	E. I.
" Canada Erigeron.	" Erigerontis.	Erig. Canadense (flowering herb).	U. S.
" Caraway.	" Cari. Sp.Junip. Co.	Carum carui (seed).	Temp. Lat. C_{10} H_{16} Carvene $C_{10}H_{14}O$ Carvol.
" Cassia.	" Cinnamomi. Aq., Sp.	Cinnamomum aromaticum (Cassia-bark).	China, etc.
" Cinnamon.	" Cinnamomi. Aq. and Sp.	Cin. zeylanicum (Ceylon cin.-bark).	Ceylon.
" Cloves.	" Caryophylli.	Eugenia caryophyl- lata(flower buds).	E. I. (Eugenic Acid or Eugenol C_{10} H_{12} O_2 Ter- pene C_{10} H_{16}.)
" Coriander.	" Coriandri.	Seeds of Corian- drum sativum.	Temp. Lat.
" Dill (anethi).		Anethum graveo- lens (fruit).	So. Eu. Asia Minor.
" Eucalyptus.	" Eucalypti.	Eucal. globulus (leaves).	Australia. Tasmania.
" Fennel.	" Fœniculi. Aq.and Sp.Jun. Co.	Fœniculum vulgare (fruit).	So. Eu. (com- position like Anise).

mon Name.	*Off. Name.*	*Botanical Source.*	*Geog. Source.*
Geranium. Rose Geranium. Roshe or Rose Oil. Gingergrass.		Andropogon schœnanthus (grass).	India (somewhat like oil of rose).
Citronella.		Androp. nardus (do.).	India.
Lemon Grass. Verbena. Indian Melissa.		Androp. citratus (do.).	(do.)
Ginger.		Zingiberis officinalis	Asia, Af., W. I. $(C_{10} H_{16} H_2 O.)$
Hedeoma. Pennyroyal.	Oleum Hedeomæ.	Hedeoma pulegioides (herb).	U. S.
Horsemint.		Monarda punctata (herb).	U. S. H. C. & Thymol.
Hyssop. Levant.		Hyssopus officinalis (herb).	So. Eu.
Wormseed.		Santonica — unexpanded flowers of Artemisia cina.	Asia.
Myrrh.		Balsamodendron myrrha.	So. Arabia.
Origanum. Sweet Marjoram.		Origanum vulgare.	Asia, Eu., U. S.
Peppermint.	" { Menthæ. Piperitæ. Aq. Sp. Troch. Pil. Rhei. Co.	Mentha Peperita (herb).	U. S. (Menthol or mint camphor. $C_{10} H_{20} O$ & $C_{10} H_{18}$).
" Chinese.			China (Menthol).
Pimento. Allspice.	" Pimentæ. Spts. Myrciæ. " Ammon. Aro.	Eugenia pimenta (fruit).	W. I., Cen. & So. Am. (Like oil cloves.)
Red Cedar.		Juniperus virginiana	N. A.
Rose.	" Rosæ.	Rosa damascena.	Turkey.
Rosemary.	" Rosmarina. Lin. Saponis. Spts. Odoratus. Tr. Lav. Co.	Rosmarinus officinalis (tops).	So. France, Italy.
Rue.	" Rutæ.	Ruta graveolens (herb).	So. Eu.
Wormwood.		Artemisia absinthium (herb).	No. Af., Eu., U.S.

Common Name.	Off. Name.	Botanical Source.	Geog. Source.
Oil of Wormseed.	Oleum Chenopodii.	Chenopodium anthelminticum (fruit)	U. S.
" Jaborandi.		Pilocarpus pennatifolius.	So.Am.(contains $C_{10}H_{16}$, &c.
" Nutmeg.	" Myristicæ. Spts. "	Kernels of fruit of Myristica fragrans.	E.&W.I.,S.A.&c. (do.)
" Parsley.		Petroselinum sativum(root & seed).	So. Eu. (do.)
" Sassafras.	" Sassafras. Tro. Cubeb.	Sassafras officinale (roots).	No. Am. (do.)
" Spearmint.	" Menthæ Viridis.Aq.Sp.	Mentha viridis (herb).	U. S. (do.)
" Thyme.	" Thymi.	Thymus vulgaris.	Eu.(do.&thymol)

CLASS 3. PRODUCED BY REACTIONS. COMPLEX.

Common Name.	Off. Name.	Botanical Source.	Geog. Source.
Oil of Birch.		Betula lenta.	U. S. (Like gaultheria.)
" Bitter Almonds.	Oleum Amygdalæ Amaræ. Aq.	Amygdalus communis (Amara) (fruit).	W. Asia.
" Gaultheria. Wintergreen. Checkerberry	Oleum Gaultheriæ. Tro.Morph.et Ipec. Spts. Gaulth.	Gaultheria procumbens.	U. S.
" Mustard.	Oleum Sinapis Volatile. Lin. Sinapis Comp.	Sinapis nigra.	Eu., As., U. S.

CLASS 4. SULPHURETTED OILS. (POLYNARY.)

Common Name.	Off. Name.	Botanical Source.	Geog. Source.
Oil of Assafœtida.		Assafœtida (Gum resin from Ferula narthex).	Asia.
" Garlic.		Allium sativum (bulb).	Temp. climes.
" Mustard.	Ol.Sinapis Volatile. Lin. Sinapis Comp.	Sinapis nigra (seed).	Eu., Asia, U. S.
" Armoracia. Horse Radish.		Cochlearia armoracia (root).	Eu. and N. Am.
" Reseda. Mignonette.		Reseda odorata (root).	Eu. and U. S.

UNCLASSED.

Common Name.	Off. Name.	Botanical Source.	Geog. Source.
Oil of Ammoniac.		Ammoniac (Gumresin from Dorema ammoniacum).	Persia, Tartary.

Common Name.	Off. Name.	Botanical Source.	Geog. Source.
Oil of Canada		Asarum canadense	N. A.
Snakeroot.		(root).	
Wild Ginger.			
" Calamus.		Acorus calamus	Eu., Asia, N. A.
Sweet-flag.		(root).	
" Cumin.		Cuminum cyminum	Egypt, So. Eu.
		(fruit).	
" Sandal.	Oleum Santali.	Santalum album	So. India and
		(wood).	E. I.
" Valerian.	" Valerianæ.	Valeriana officinalis	Eu. and U. S.
		(root).	

The following drugs depend principally upon volatile oils for medicinal action. They are best used in infusion. They may be made into fl. exts. by repercolation. Alcoholic menstrua.

Common Name.	Off. Name.	Botanical Source.	Geog. Source.
Horse Balm.		Collinsonia canadensis(herb).	N. A.
Buchu.	Buchu. Fl. Ext.	Barosma betulina. B. crenulata. B. serratifolia (leaves).	So. Af.
Summer Savory.		Satureja hortensis.	So. Eu.
Yerba Buena.		Micromeria Douglassii.	Cal., Utah.
Masterwort.		Imperatoria ostruthium.	So. and Cen. Eu.
Orris root. ·		Iris. Flor. (root).	Eu.
{ Laurel. { Sweet Bay.		Laurus nobilis (leaves and fruit).	Eu.
{ Water Cress. { Nasturtium.		Nasturtium officinale (plant).	Eu., Asia, Am.
Elder-flowers.	Sambucus.	Samb. canadensis.	N. Am.
Goldenrod.		Solidago odora.	U. S.
Tansy.	Tanacetum.	Tanacet. vulgare.	U. S.

REACTIONARY DRUGS.

CLASS 1. PRODUCING H. CY. BY REACTION BETWEEN AMYGDALIN AND EMULSION.

Common Name.	Off. Name.	Botanical Source.	Geog. Source.
Bitter Almonds. (Cont.Am.and Em.)	Amygdala Amara. Off. in Syr. Am.	Amygdalus communis (amara).	So. W. Eu.

Common Name.	Off. Name.	Botanical Source.	Geog. Source.
Sweet Almonds.	Amygdala Dulcis.	Amygdalus com-	Jordan, Malaga
(Cont. Emulsin.)	Syr. and Mist.	munis (dulcis).	= Hard-shelled.
			Valencia = Soft-shelled.
Cherry Laurel.		Prunus lauro-	Asia and Eu.
(Aq. Lauro-cerasi.)		cerasus.	
Peach meats.		Amygdalus persica.	Temp. climes.
Wild Cherry.	Prunus Virginiana.	Cerasus serotina	N. Am.
Black "	Inf., Syr., Fl. Ext.	(bark).	

H Cy. produced in conjunction with oil of bitter almonds.

Cyanogen, the acid radical, exists in H Cy and all cyanides (as K Cy); in cyanates (K Cy O); in cyanurets (as $K_3 Cy_3 O_3$); in fulminates ($K_2 Cy_2 O_2$); in sulphocyanides (K Cy S); in ferrocyanides ($K_4 Fe'' Cy_6$); in ferricyanides ($K_3 Fe''' Cy_6$); nitro-prussides ($Na_2 (NO) Fe'' Cy_5$).

H Cy, off., as Acidum Hydrocyanicum Dilutum, obtained by distilling $K_4 Fe'' Cy_6 + H_2 SO_4$ or by mixing Ag Cy with II Cl. Off. strength 2%.

CLASS 2. PRODUCING OIL OF WINTERGREEN (METHYL-SALICYLATE.)

Common Name.	Off. Name.	Botanical Name.	Geog. Source.
Gaultheria.	Gaultheria.	Gaultheria pro-	No. Am.
Dewberry.	Syr. Sars. Co.	cumbens (leaves).	
Boxberry.			
Teaberry.			
Checkerberry.			
Wintergreen.			
Black Birch.		Betula lenta (bark	No. Am.
Cherry "		and leaves) (gaul-	
Sweet "		therin and un-	
		known ferment).	

Of kindred character are :—

Meadow Sweet.		Spirea ulmaria.	Eu.
Heliotrope.		Heliotropium	In., Eu., Am.
		corymbosum.	

Salicylic Acid, from Indigo, Salicin, Populin, etc., by treating with fused K HO.

Also, carbolic acid neutralized with Na HO, the carbolate of sodium dried, heated and treated with dry CO_2 to form Na_2 Sal., $Na_2 CO_3$ and free carbolic acid. Na_2 Sal. decomposed with H Cl. and the Sal. Acid purified by dialysis.

CLASS 3. PRODUCING ACRID OILS.

Common Name.	Off. Name.	Botanical Source.	Geog. Source.
White Mustard.	Sinapis alba.	Sinapis alba (seed).	So. Eu., U. S., W. Asia.

The glucoside Sinalbin + (ferment) myrosin, = Sinapina.
Bisulphate (Vol. Alk.) + glucose + Acrinyl Sulphocyanate.

Common Name.	Off. Name.	Botanical Source.	Geog. Source.
Black Mustard.	Sinapis nigra. Chart. Sinapis.	Sinapis nigra (seed).	So. Eu., W. Asia, U. S.

Sinnigrin (the glucoside myromic acid and potassium)+(ferment) myrosin = *Volatile Oil of Mustard* (Allyl Sulphocyanide $C_3 H_5 CNS$), etc.

Horse Radish.	Cochlearia armor-acia (root).	Eu., U. S.
Mignonette.	Reseda odorata (root).	Eu., U. S.
Shepherd's Purse.	Capsella bursa-pastoris.	Eu.
Cress.	Lepidum sativum, etc.	Eu. and Am.
Bitter Candytuft.	Iberis amara.	Eu. and Am.

Also the wild mustard and the radishes.

DRUGS CONTAINING VOLATILE OIL AND RESIN.

CLASS 1. AROMATICS PROPER.

Common Name.	Officinals.	Botanical Source.	Geog. Source.
Benzoin. Spice bush.		Benzoinum odori-ferum (bark and fruit).	Can. and U. S.
Canada Snake-root. Wild Ginger.		Asarum canadense (rhizome & rootlets).	" "
Calamus. Sweet Flag.	Calamus. Fl. Ext., Vin. Rhei.	Acorus calamus (root).	N.Am.,N.Asia.
Canella. Whitewood. Wild Cinnamon.		Canella alba (bark).	W. I.
Cascarilla.	Cascarilla.	Croton eluteria (bark).	"
Cloves.	Caryophyllus. Tr. Rhei. Aro., Vin. Opii. Syr. Rhei. Aro., Tr. Lav. Co.	Eugenia caryophyl-lata (unexpanded flowers).	E. I., W. I., etc.
Cardamom.*	Cardamomum. Tr.Card.,Tr. Rhei., " " Co., " " Dulcis. Vin. Aloes, Pv. Aromat., Ext. Coloc. Co., Tr. Gent. Co.	Elettaria Carda-momum (fruit).	India.

* Contains no resin, but contains fixed oil.

Common Name.	Officinals.	Botanical Source.	Geog. Source.
Cinnamon Ceylon.	Cinnamomum. Tr. Cinnam.,	Cinnamomum. Zeylanicum.	Ceylon.
Do., Chinese. Cassia.	Pv. Arom., Tr. Rhei. Aro., Tr. Lav. Co., Syr. Rhei. Aro., Tr. Catechu Co.	Cin. aromaticum (inner bark).	China.
Ginger.	Zingiberis. Tinct. Zing., Fl. Ext. " Troch. " Oleores " Syr. " Acid Sul. Aro., Vin. Aloes, Pv. Arom., Pv. Rhei. Co.	Zingiberis officinale (root).	Asia., E. and W. I.
Liatris. Deer's tongue.		Liatris odoratissima (root and leaves).	N. A.
Mace.	Macis.	Arillus of Nutmeg.	E. and W. I., So. Am.
Mountain Balm. Consumptive's Weed.		Eriodyction califor- nicum (leaves).	Cal.
Nutmeg.*	Myristica. Tr. Rhei. Aro., Pv. Aromat., Syr. Rhei. Aro., Tr. Lav. Co., Troch. Mag., Troch. Sod. Bicarb. Acet. Opii.	Myristica fragrans (kernel of seed).	E. and W. I., So. Am.
Pimento. Allspice.	Pimenta.	Eugenia pimenta (unripe berries).	W. I., Cent. Am., etc.
Sassafras.	Sassafras. Dec. Sars. Co., Syr. " " Fl. Ext. " "	Sassafras officinalis (bark of root).	U. S.

CLASS 2. CONTAIN VOL. OIL AND PUNGENT RESIN.

Common Name.	Officinals.	Botanical Source.	Geog. Source.
Cubebs.	Cubeba. Tinct., Fl. Ext., Troch., Oleoresin.	Cubeba officinalis (Piper Cubeba) unripe fruit.	E. I.
Cypripedium. Ladies Slipper. American Valerian.	Cypripedium. Fl. Ext.	Cypripedium pu- bescens (root).	Can. and U. S

* Contains no resin, but contains fixed oil.

Common Name.	Officinals.	Botanical Source.	Geog. Source.
Grindelia.	Grindelia.	Grindelia robusta	California, etc.
Resin leaf.	Fl. Ext.	(leaves and tops).	
Levisticum.		Ligusticum levis-	So. Eu.
Lovage.		ticum (root).	
Pepper.	Piper.	Piper nigrum	E. and W. I.
	Oleoresin.	(unripe berries).	

CLASS 3. CONTAIN VOL. OIL AND ACRID RESIN.

Common Name.	Officinals.	Botanical Source.	Geog. Source.
Alisma.		Alisma plantago	Eu. and N. Am.
Water Plantain.		(rhizome).	
Anacardium.		Anacardium occi-	Tropical Am.,
Cashew Nut.		dentale (fruit).	Eu., Af.
Arnica Flowers.	Arnicæ Flores.	Arnica montana.	Eu.
	Tinct. Arnicæ Florum.		
Arnica Root.	Arnicæ Radix.	do.,	do.
	Tinct., Ext., Fl.Ext., Emp.		
Arum.		Arisæma or Arum	N. Am.
Indian Turnip.		triphyllum (tuber).	
Asclepias.		Asclepias incarnata	Can., U. S.
Flesh colored.		(rhizome & rootlets).	
Pleurisy Root.	Asclepias.	Asclepias tuberosa	U. S.
		(root).	
Armoracia.		Cochlearia armor-	Eu. and Am.
Horse Radish.		acia (root).	
Bursa Pastoris.		Bursa pastoris.	Eu.
Shepherd's Purse.			
American Canna-	Cannabis Amer-	Cannabis sativa	So. U. S.
bis.	icana.	(flowering tops).	
Indian Cannabis.	Cannabis Indica. Ext., Fl. Ext., Tinct.	Can. sativa (flowering tops of female plant).	E. I.
Dracontium.		Dracontium fœti-	N. Am.
Skunk Cabbage.		dum, Ictodes fœtidus (root).	
Galangal.		Alpinia officinarum	So. China.
East Indian Catarrh Root.		(rhizome).	
Glechoma.		Glechoma heder-	Eu., N. A.
Ground Ivy.		acea (leaves).	
Heracleum.		Heracleum lanatum	U. S.
Cow-parsnip.		(root, leaves and	
Masterwort.		fruit).	
Inula.	Inula.	Inula helenium	Asia. U. S.
Elecampane.		(root).	

Common Name.	Officinals.	Botanical Source.	Geog. Source.
Matico (Leaves).	Matico. Fl. Ext., Tinct.	Artanthe elongatai. Piper angustifolium.	Trop. Am.
Myrica. Bayberry bark. Wax Myrtle.		Myrica cerifera.	New Eng.
Pellitory.	Pyrethrum. Tinct.	Anacyclus pyrethrum (root).	N. W. Af.
Persian Insect Powder Flowers. Dalmation do.		Pyrethrum roseum and carneum. Pyreth cinerariæ- folium.	W. Asia. Dalmatia.
Para-cress. Spilanthes.		Spilanthes oleracea (herb).	So. Am., India.
Prickly Ash. Toothache tree. Angelica " Suterberry.	Xanthoxylum. Fl. Ext.	Xanthoxylum fraxineum. X. carolinianum (bark).	N. A.
Winter's Bark. Wintera.		Drimy's Winteri.	So. Am.
Zedoary.		Curcuma zedoaria (rhizome).	Ind. & E. I.
Paradise Seed. Guinea Grains. Malegueta pepper		Amomum granum-paradisi.	W. Af.

DRUGS CONTAINING VOL. OIL, BITTER-PRINCIPLE AND EXTRACTIVE.

Mostly aromatic, bitter drugs, consequently both tonic and stimulant. Some contain tannin enough to render them astringent. Some, as hops, lupulin, serpentaria, scutellaria, valerian and cimicifuga, are sedative. They yield much of their activity to boiling water, and are adapted to infusion. Alcohol sp. gr. 835 best general menstruum for Fl. Ext. Repercolation best method.

Common Name.	Officinals.	Botanical Source.	Geog. Source.
Absinthium. Wormwood.	Absinthium. Vin. Arom.	Artemisia absinth- ium (leaves&tops)	N. Af., Eu. As., U. S.
Southernwood. Old Man. Boy's-love.		Artemisia abrota- num (herb).	do.
Mugwort.		Artemisia vulgaris (herb).	do.
Tarragon.		Art. dracunculus.	Siberia, Tart. & So. Eu.
Roman Wormwood.		Art. ponticum.	do. & U. S.

Common Name.	Officinals.	Botanical Source.	Geog. Source.
Yarrow.		Achillea millefolium (herb).	Am., Eu.
Ailanthus. Tree of Heaven. Chinese Sumach.		Ailanthus glandulosa (bark).	China, Eu., U. S.
Ragweed.		Ambrosia trifida (herb).	N. Am.
Hogweed.		Amb. artemisiæfolia (herb).	N. Am.
Angelica.		Archangelica atropurpurea (root). Arch. officinalis (root).	N. Am. Eu.
Angustura.		Galipea cusparia (bark).	So. Am.
Chamomile. (English.)	Anthemis.	Anthemis nobilis (flowers).	So. & W. Eu.
Chamomile. (German.)	Matricaria.	Matricaria chamomilla (herb).	Eu.
False Sarsaparilla.		Aralia nudicaulis (root).	Can. & U. S.
Aralia bark.		Aralia spinosa (bark).	So. U. S.
Bitter Orange-peel.	Aurantii Amari Cortex. Tr. Aur. Am., Fl., Ext. " " Tr. Gent. Co., " Cinch. Co.	Citrus vulgaris (rind).	E. & W. I., So. Eu., etc.
Calendula. Marigold.	Calendula. Tinct. Calend.	Calendula officinalis (flowering herb).	So. Eu.
Carthamus (?) Safflower. Am. Saffron.		Carthamus tinctorius (florets).	Eu.
Catnep. Catmint.		Nepeta cataria (herb).	As., Eu., U. S.
Cotula. Mayweed.		Maruta or Anthemis cotula (herb).	Eu. & N. Am.
Crocus. Saffron.	Crocus. Tinct. Croci.	Crocus sativus (stigmas).	Eu. & U. S.
Fleabane Erigeron.		Erig. heterophyllum " Philadelphicum (leaves and tops).	Can. & U. S.
Canada fleabane. " Erigeron.		Erigeron canadense.	N. Am.
Life Everlasting. Gnaphalium.		Different species of Gnaphalium.	Eu. & U. S.

Common Name.	Officinals.	Botanical Source.	Geog. Source.
Hops. -	Humulus. Tinct. Humuli.	Humulus lupulus (strobiles).	Temp. climes.
Hypericum. St. John's Wort.		Hypericum perforatum (herb).	Eu., N. Af., U. S.
Iberis (cont. sulph. oil and amorph. bit. prin. Lepidin).		Lepidium iberis (plant).	S. E. Siberia.
Leonorus. Motherwort.		Leonorus cardiaca (herb).	Eu., N. As., N. Am.
Leptandra. Culver's-root. Black-root.	Leptandra. Ext. and Fl. Ext.	Leptandra virginica (root and rootlets). Bit. prin. cryst. glucoside.	Can., U. S.
Lupulin (bit. prin. lupamaric acid).	Lupulinum. Fl. Ext.,Oleoresin,	Glandular powder from hops.	Temp. climes.
Lycopus. Bugleweed.		Lycopus virginicus (herb).	Can. & U. S.
Magnolia. Sweet Bay. Beaver tree. Swamp Sassafras.	Magnolia.	Magnolia glauca (bark).	East. U. S.
Horehound. (Cryst. bit. prin.)	Marrubium.	Marrubium vulgare (herb).	As., Eu., Am.
Origanum. Wild Marjoram.	Origanum. Vin. Arom.	Origanum vulgare (herb).	do.
Parthenium. Feverfew.		Pyrethrum parthenium (herb).	Eu.
Bitter Polygala. " Milkwort.		Polygala rubella (herb).	U. S.
Black Snakeroot. " Cohosh. Cimicifuga.	Cimicifuga. Fl. Ex., Tinct.	Cimicifuga racemosa (root and rootlets).	Can. & U. S.
Juniper berries.	Juniperus.	Juniperus communis (fruit).	Eu. & Am.
Santonica. Levant Wormseed.	Santonica. Source of Santonin.	Unexpanded flowers of Artemisia cina.	As.
Sage.	Salvia. Vin. Arom.	Salvia officinalis (herb).	U. S.
Skullcap.	Scutellaria. Fl. Ext.	Scutellaria lateriflora (herb).	N. Am.
Savine (?).	Sabina. Fl. Ext., Cerate.	Tops of Juniperus sabina.	Eu., Am.
Serpentaria. Virginia Snake-root.	Serpentaria. Fl. Ext., Tinct., Tr. Cinch. Co.	Aristolochia serpentaria (root).	U. S.
Simaruba.		Sim. officinalis (bark of root).	S. Am.

Common Name.	Officinals.	Botanical Source.	Geog. Source.
Pinkroot. Spigelia. Maryland Pink. Worm-grass.	Spigelia. Fl. Ext.	Spigelia marilandica (root).	U. S.
Valerian (Eng.).	Valeriana. El. Ext.,	Valeriana officinalis (root).	Eu., U. S.
Teucrium. Germander.	Tr. Val., Tr. Val. Am., Abs. Val.	Different varieties Teucrium.	Eu.

NATURAL OLEORESINS AND KINDRED BODIES
OR DERIVATIVES.

Common Name.	Officinals.	Botanical Source.	Geog. Source.
Turpentine. Common Frank- incense. White Pitch.	Terebinthina. Emp. Galbani.	Pinus palustris, etc.	So. U. S.
Tar.	Pix Liquida. Syrup and Ungt.	do. By dest. dist.	do.
Hemlock-pitch. Canada-pitch.	Pix Canadensis. Emp. Picis Can.	Abies canadensis.	No. U. S. & Can.
Burgundy "	Pix Burgundica. Emp. Picis Burg., " " Cum. Canth., Emp. Ferri., Emp. Gal- bani, Emp. Opii.	Abies excelsa.	Eu.
Fir-Balsam. Canada-balsam. Can. Turpentine.	Terebinthina Canadensis. Charta Canth. Collod. Flexile.	Abies balsamea.	No. U. S. & Can.
Venice " Terebinthina Ve- neta.		Larix Europœa.	So. & S.W. Eu.
Chian Turp.		Pistacia terebinthus.	Scio., So. Eu.
Mastic.	Mastiche. Pil. Aloes et Ma- stiches.	" lentiscus.	do. & E. I.
Olibanum. Indian Frankin- cense.		Boswellia Carterii.	So. Arabia.
Copaiva.	Copaiba. Massa Copaibæ.	Copaifera Langs dorfii, etc.	So. Am.
Amber. Succinum.		Coniferæ, now ex- tinct (?).	So. E. Eu.

Common Name.	Officinals.	Botanical Source.	Geog. Source.
Strassburg Turp.		Abies pectinata.	Eu.
Hungarian "		Pinus pumilio.	Eu.
Carama.		Icica carama.	Cent. & S. Am.
Tacamahaca.		Elaphruim tomento-	So. Am.
		sum, &c.	
Anime.			So. India.
Spruce Gum.		Abies Nigra & Abies	No. Am.
		Alba.	

DERIVATIVES AND ALLIED BODIES.

From Turpentine—Oleum Terebinthinæ (off.) (Lin. Canth. and Lin. Tereb.) Resina (off.) (Ceratum Resinæ, Emp. Resinæ, etc.)

From Canada-pitch—or from branches of tree Abies Canadensis—Oil of Hemlock or Oil of Spruce.

From Fir-balsam—Oil of Fir.

From Copaiva—Oleum Copaibæ (off.), Resina Copaibæ (off.).

From *Wood Tar*, subjected to distillation.

Light Oil of Wood Tar—Acetic Acid, Acetone, Methylic-alcohol, Toluol, Xylol, Cumol, Eupion, etc.

Heavy Oil of Wood Tar—Creasotum (a complex body), small quantities of Carbolic Acid, Naphthalin, Paraffin, etc. (Aq. Creasoti, off.).

Residue—Black-pitch.

From *Coal Tar*, separated in hydraulic main.

Light Oil of Coal Tar—Benzole, Toluol, Xylol, Cumol, etc.

Heavy Oil of Coal Tar—Cresylic Acid, Naphthalin, Anilin, Paraffin, etc., etc., and Acidum Carbolicum (off.) (Ungt. Acid. Carbol.).

Residue—Coal-Tar pitch, asphalt.

From Crude Petroleum—Rock Oil.

Rhigolene, Gasoline, C. B. A. Naphthas, (Benzinum off.) Kerosene, Heavier Paraffins (Spindle Oil, Vaseline, Cosmoline, Deodoraline, Paraffin Wax), etc., etc., and Petrolatum (off.).

From Amber,—Oil of Amber—Succinic Acid.

RESINS, GUM RESINS AND BALSAMS.

Resins.—When pure, mostly brittle solids, softening by heat; not vólatile; mostly heavier than water; but little soluble in water; soluble in alcohol, ether, benzole, chloroform and volatile oils; many soluble in aqueous alkalies.

Gum Resins.—Resins associated with gum. Separated by fusion and use of proper solvents.

Oleoresins.—Resins associated with volatile oils. Separated by distillation with water.

Balsams.—Oleoresins associated with benzoic or cinnamic acids.

Alcohol, menstruum for tinctures or fluid extracts. Incompatible with Aquæ, Decocta, Infusa, etc.

Common Name.	Officinals.	Botanical Source.	Geog. Source.
Peru Balsam.	Balsamum Peruvianum.	Myroxylon Pareiræ.	Cent. Am.
Tolu "	Balsamum Tolutanum. Tr. Tolu and Syr. Tolu.	Myroxylon toluifera.	So. Am., Colombia.
Benzoin.	Benzoinum. Adeps Benz ,Tinct. and Co. Tinct.	Styrax benzoin.	Borneo, Sumatra, Siam,&c.
Storax.	Styrax. Tr. Benz. Co.	Liquidamber orientalis.	S. W. Asia Minor.
Balm of Gilead Buds. Poplar "		Populus balsamifera or candicus.	U. S.
Sweet Gum. Liquidamber.		Liquidamber styraciflua.	N. Am., So. U. S.

GUM RESINS.

Common Name.	Officinals.	Botanical Source.	Geog. Source.
Guaiac.			
Lignum-vitæ Resin. Tree of Life "	Guaiaci Resina. Tr. and Am. Tr. Pil. Ant. Co.	Guaiacum officinale.	W. I., San Domingo, Hayti.(?)
Gamboge.	Cambogia. Pil. Cath. Co.	Garcinia Hamburii.	Siam,Campodia, Cochin China.
Scammony.	Scammonium. Resina Scammonii.	Convolvulus scammonia.	Asia Minor. Greece.
Myrrh.	Myrrha.Tr. Myrrh., Tr. Al. and Myrrh., Pil. " " Mist. Ferri Co. Pil. " " " Galbani " " Rhei "	Balsamodendron myrrha.	E. Africa. Arabia.
True Balm of Gilead. Opobalsamum.		Allied Species.	do.
Bdellium.		" "	W. Africa.
Ammoniac.	Ammoniacum. Emp. Am., Emp. Am. c̄ Hyd. Mist. Am.	Dorema ammoniacum.	Persia and Tartary.

Common Name.	Officinals.	Botanical Source.	Geog. Source.
Galbanum.	Galbanum. Pil. Galb. Co. Emp. Galb.	Ferula galbaniflua.	N. Persia.
Asafetida.	Asafœtida. Emp. Asafœt. Tr. Asaf., Mist. Asaf. Mist. Mag. et Asaf., Emp. Asaf., Pil. Asaf., Pll. Al. and Asaf., Pil. Galbani Co.	Ferula narthex.	Persia, Afghanistan.
Euphorbium.		Euphorbia resinifera.	Atlas Mts., Morocco.
Opopanax.		Opopanax chironium.	So. Europe.
Sagapenum.		Some variety of Ferula.	Persia.
Hedera. Ivy Gum.		Hedera helix.	Levant, So. Europe.

RESINS AND RESINOUS DRUGS OWING THEIR ACTIVITY TO RESINS.

Common Name.	Officinals.	Botanical Source.	Geog. Source.
Agaric Alba. White Agaric.		Fungus growing on Larch trees.	Cent. and So. Eu., W. Asia.
Koosso. Cusso. Kousso.	Brayera. Fl. Ext. Bray. Infus. "	Brayera anthelmintica. (Female inflorescence.)	Abyssinia.
Blue Cohosh. Squaw-root. Pappoose-root.	Caulophyllum.	Caulophyllum thalictroides (rhizome)	U. S.
Wild Ipecac. Large flowering Spurge.		Euphorbia corollata (root).	U. S.
Carolina Ipecac. Ipecac Spurge.		Euphorbia ipecacuanha (root).	U. S.
Cotton Root Bark.	Gossypii Radicis Cortex. Fl. Ext.	Gossypium herbaceum (bark).	Sub-tropical climates.
Jalap.	Jalapa. Resin, Abstract, Pulv. Jalap. Co.	Exogonium purga (tuber).	Mexico.
Man-root. Wild Jalap. " Potato.		Ipomœa pandurata (tuber).	U. S.
Turpeth root.		Ipomœa turpethum (root).	India.
Labdanum.		Cistus creticus (resin).	Greece and Levant.

Common Name.	Officinals.	Botanical Source.	Geog. Source.
Lacca. Stick-lac. Seed-lac. Grain-lac. Shellac.		Resin produced by punctures of insects, Coccus lacca.	E. I.
Mezereum.	Mezereum. Fl. Ex. Mezerei, Ungt. " Ext. " Dec. Sars. Co. Fl.Ext. " " Lin.Sinapis "	Daphne mezereum. " laureola,etc. (bark).	Europe, Asia Minor.
Mandrake.	Podophyllum. Abstract Podoph. Ext. Podoph. Res. " Fl. Ext. "	Podophyllum pellatum (rhizome and rootlets).	U. S.
Dragon's Blood. Resina Draconis.		Calamus draco. (Climbing Palm.) (Resin exudes upon fruit.)	E. I., Borneo, Sumatra.
Kameela. Kamala. Rottlera.	Kamala.	Mallotus philippinensis (powder and hairs from capsules).	Australia, E. China, So. Arabia, India.
Thapsia.		Thapsia garganica.	So. Europe, N. Africa.
Elemi.		Derived from different botanical sources.	Mexico, Manila, Brazil, etc.
Sandarac.		Callitris quadrivalvis.	N.W. Africa.

ALKALOIDAL DRUGS.

An Alkaloid is one of a group of organic bodies containing Nitrogen, their solutions having an alkaline reaction, capable of uniting with acids to form salts. Or, Alkaloids are alkali-like bodies, containing Nitrogen, *mostly* of vegetable origin, usually the active principle of the drug furnishing them, often dangerous poisons, general antidotes to which are emetics and strong astringents, as tannic acid, strong tea, coffee, etc. They are usually little soluble in water, but are soluble in alcohol ; have bitter taste, no odor. They are ppt. by tannin, mercuric chloride, auric chloride, picric acid, phosphomolybdic acid, phosphotungstic acid, solution of iodine and potassic iodide, etc. Estimated by ppt. by tannin, triturating moist ppt. with $Pb. CO_3$, drying, extracting with alcohol, chloroform, ether, etc., and evaporating solvents. Also, by agitating acid and alkaline solutions successively with alcohol, chloroform, ether, benzole, etc., and evaporating solvents.

Common Name and Botanical and Geog. Source.	Officinals.	Alkaloids.	Doses and Uses.
Aconite Root. " Leaves. [Aconitum napellus.] Asia and Europe.	Aconitum (root). Abst. Aconiti. Ext. " " " Fluidum. Tinct. "	Napellina, Aconella, Lycotonina, Pseudaconitia. Aconitina or Aconitia.*	Petit's $\frac{1}{200}$ gr.* Duquesnel's $\frac{1}{125}$ grain. Merck's, from Himalaya Root, $\frac{1}{100}$ gr. Merck's *common* $\frac{1}{10}$ grain. Freidlander's (?) $\frac{1}{2}$ gr.
Akazga Bark. Boundou. Ikaja. [Unknown variety of Strychnos.] West Africa.		Akazgina.	Like Strychnina.
Alstonia. Dita Bark. [Alstonia scholaris.] Philippine Islands.		Ditamina.	Bitter tonic and intermittent.
Andira. Cabbage Tree Bark. [Andira inermis.] W. I. and So. Am.		Jamaicina. Lurinamina.	Identical with Berberina.
Antiaris. [Gum resin from Antiaris toxicaria, the Upas tree.] Java.		Antiarina.	Dangerous poison. Like physostigmina or eserina. Dose, $\frac{1}{65}$ to $\frac{1}{12}$ grain.
Argemone. Prickly Poppy. [Argemone Mexicana.] Mex. and W. I.		Morphina.	
Baptisia. Wild Indigo. [Baptisia tinctoria.] (Tops and bark.) New Eng.		Baptisina.	Emetic Bitter.
Belladonna. Deadly Nightshade. [Atropa belladonna.] (Root and leaves.) Eu. and U. S.	Belladonnæ Folia. Ext. Bell. Alc. Tinct. " Ungt. " Belladonnæ Radix. Abs.Bell., Emp.Bell. Ext. " Fl.,Lin. " Atropina and Atropinæ Sulph.	Atropina.	Stimulant Narcotic, Antispasmodic. Dose, $\frac{1}{100}$ to $\frac{1}{25}$ grain.
Barberry Bark. [Berberis vulgaris.] As., Eu. and Am.		Berberina.	Alterative tonic. 2 to 5 grains.

Common Name and Botanical and Geog. Source.	Officinals.	Alkaloids.	Doses and Uses.
Boldo Leaves. [Peumus boldus.] Chili.		Boldina.	Bitter tonic and stimulant.
Coffee (fruit). [Caffea arabica.] Af., So. Am., etc.	Caffeina.	Caffeina.	Nervous stimulant and sedative. Dose, ½ gr.
Columbo root. [Jateorrhiza calumba,] E. Africa.	Columba. Ext. Columb. Fl. Tinct. "	Berberina. (Columbin (?), a neutral principle.)	Bitter tonic.
Cayenne Pepper. [Capsicum fastigiatum.]	Capsicum. Ext. Capsici Fl. Oleores. " Tinct. "	(Said to contain a volatile alkaloid. Its acridity due to capsaicin, which is a neut. prin.)	Stimulant.
Celandine. [Chelidonium majus.] Eu., U. S.	Chelidonium.	Chelidonina. { Chelerythrina { or Pyrrhopina.	Acrid Narcotic.
Cicuta. Water Hemlock. [Cicuta virosa.] (Herb and root.) America.		Cicutina. (Vol. Alkaloid.)	Acrid Narcotic.
Conium. Spotted Hemlock. [Conium maculatum.] (Fruit.) Temp. latitudes.	Conium (fruit). Abst., Alc. Ext., Fl. Ext., Tinct.	Conina. Vol. Alk.	Narcotic. Dose, 1/20 to 1/10 gr.
Goldthread. [Coptis trifolia.] (Plant.) America.		Berberina. Coptina.	Bitter tonic.
Cinchona. Peruvian Bark. Jesuit's Bark. So Am. and India.	Cinchona. Infus. Cinchonæ. Cinchonidinæ Sulph. Cinchonina. Cinchoninæ Sulph. Quinidinæ Sulph. Quinina. Quininæ Bisulph. Quininæ Hydrobromas. Quininæ Hydrochloras. Quininæ Sulphas. " Valerianas.	Quinina. Quinidina. Quinicina. Paytayina. Cusconina, etc. Cinchonina. Cinchonidina. Cinchonicina.	Tonic, febrifuge. Dose, 1 to 10 grs. Dose, 2 to 20 grs.

Common Name and Botanical and Geog. Source.	Officinals.	Alkaloids.	Doses and Uses.
Calisaya Bark. [Cinchona calisaya.] Red Bark. [Cinchona succirubra.]	Cinchona Flava. Ext., Fl. Ext., Tinct. Cinchona Rubra. Tinct. Cinchon. Comp.		
Colchicum. Meadow Saffron. [Colchicum autumnale.] (Corm.) (Seed.) Europe.	Colchici Radix. Ext. Colch. Rad. " " " Fl. Vin. " " Colchici Semen. Ext. Colch. Sem. Fl. Tinct. " " Vin. " "	Colchicina.	Narcotic, diuretic. Dose, $\frac{1}{400}$ to $\frac{1}{100}$ grain. Dose of drug, 2 to 8 grains.
Corydalis. Turkey Corn. [Dicentra canadensis.] (Tubers.) N. America.		Corydalina. (Amorphous.)	Tonic, diuretic, alterative. Dose of drug, 10 to 30 grains.
Curare. Wourari, etc. So. Am. Arrow Poison. (Prepared from a variety of Strychnos, etc.)		Curarina.	Antispasmodic, and powerful nervous sedative. Dose of drug, $\frac{1}{10}$ grain. Dose of Alkaloid, $\frac{1}{100}$ to $\frac{1}{30}$ grain.
Larkspur Seed. [Delphinium consolida.] Eu. and U. S.		Delphinina. Staphisaina.	Acrid, narcotic poison. Dose, $\frac{1}{4}$ gr. Used mostly externally.
Duboisia. [Duboisia myoporoides.] (Leaves). Australia.		Duboisina.	Like Atropina. Dose $\frac{1}{60}$ grain.
Bittersweet. [Solanum dulcamara.] (Young branches.) Eu. and U. S.	Dulcamara. Ext. Dulc. Fl.	Solanina. (?) (May be a glucoside.) Dulcamarin is a glucoside.	Tonic-sedative.
Sassy Bark. Mancona Bark. [Erythrophlœum. guineense.] Cent. and W. Af.		Erythrophlœina. (Crystalline.)	Acrid narcotic.
Coca Leaves. [Erythroxylon coca.] So. Am.	Erythroxylon. Fl. Ext.	Cocaina. (Crystalline.) Hygrina. (Volatile.)	Diuretic, stimulant. Resembles tea and coffee. Dose of Cocaina $\frac{1}{4}$ to 1 grain.

47

Common Name and Botanical and Geog. Source.	Officinals.	Alkaloids.	Doses and Uses.
Fumitory. [Fumaria officinalis.] (Plant.) Europe.		Fumarina. (Crystalline.)	Tonic and diuretic. (Like dandelion.)
Yellow Jasmine. [Gelsemium sempervirens.] (Root.) So. U. S.	Gelsemium. Fl. Ext. and Tinct.	Gelseminina. (Like Aconitina in action.)	Arterial sedative. Dose $\frac{1}{60}$ grain.
Guarana. Paullinia. A paste from seeds of Paullinia sorbilis. So. Am.	Guarana. Fl. Ext.	Caffeina. (Yields 5%.)	Cerebral stimulant. Dose of drug 10 to 60 grs.
Goldenseal. [Hydrastis canadensis.] (Rhizome and rootlets.) Can. and U. S.	Hydrastis. Fl. Ext. and Tinct.	Hydrastina. (White.) Berberina. (Yellow.)	Astringent, tonic.
Henbane. [Hyoscyamus niger.] (Leaves.) Eu., U.S., etc.	Hyoscyamus. Abst.,Ext.Hyos.Alc., Ext.Hyos. Fl.,Tinct. Hyoscyaminæ Sulph.	Hyoscyamina.	Narcotic. $\frac{1}{50}$ to $\frac{1}{14}$ grain.
Cassena. Yaupon [Ilex cassine.] So. U. S.		Caffeina. (0.122 %.)	
Ignatia. [Strychnos ignatii.] Bean of St. Ignatius. (Seeds.) Phil. Is. and Cochin China.	Ignatia. Abst. Ignatiae. Tinct. "	Strychnina. Brucina.	Nervous stimulant. Irritant-poison. Dose, Strych., $\frac{1}{50}$ to $\frac{1}{20}$ gr. Dose, Brucia, $\frac{1}{4}$ to 1 gr.
Ipecac. [Cephælis ipecacuanha.] (Root.) So. Am.	Ipecacuanha. Ext. Ipecac. Fl. Pv. " et Opii. Tinct. " " Troch. " " Morph. et Ipecac. Syrup Ipecac., Vinum "	Emetina. (1 to 2 %.)	Emetic in dose of $\frac{1}{2}$ to $\frac{1}{4}$ grain. Diaphoretic in dose of $\frac{1}{120}$ to $\frac{1}{30}$ gr.
Laburnum. Bean Trefoil. [Cytisus laburnum.] (Bark and seeds.) So. Eu.		Citysina. (Crystalline.)	Acrid, bitter, sedative. Dose, $\frac{1}{4}$ grain.

Common Name and Botanical and Geog. Source.	Officinals.	Alkaloids.	Doses and Uses.
Culver's Root. Black Root. [Leptandra virginica.] (Rhizome and rootlets.) Can. and U. S.	Leptandra. Ext. and Fl. Ext.	Said to yield a small % of a vol. alk. not named.	Drug is an alt. cath. Dose, 20 to 60 grains. Dose of Resinoid, 1 to 4 grs.
Matrimony Vine. [Lycium vulgare.] (Bark and leaves.) So. Eu.		Lycina.	Cathartic.
Yellow Parilla. Can. Moonseed. [Menispermum canadense. (Rhizome.) N. Am.	Menispermum.	Berberina. (Yellow.) Menispermina. (?) (White.)	Tonic Alt. Diuretic.
Daffodil. [Narcissus pseudonarcissus.] (Bulb and flowers.) So. Eu.		Alakloid not named. Resembles Atropia.	Drug is Emetic, Purgative, Narcotic.
Nectandra. Bebeeru Bark. [Nectandra Rodiæi.] Br. Guiana.		Berberina. { Yellow—impure. { White—pure.	Bitter tonic, ½ to 3 grains. Drug —astringent.
Nux Vomica. Poison Nut. Quaker Buttons. [Strychnos nux Vomica.] (Seed.) E. India.	Nux Vomica. Abst.,Ext.,Fl.Ext., Tinct., Strychnina, Ferri et Strych.Cit., Syr. Ferri Quin. et Strych Phos., Strych. Sulph.	Strychnina. Brucina. Igasurina.	Nerv. stim. Irritant poison. Dose, Strych., $\frac{1}{60}$ to $\frac{1}{20}$ grs. Dose, Brucia, ¼ to 1 gr.
Oleander. [Nerium oleander.] (Leaves.) So. Eu., N. Af., W. As.		Pseudo-curarina. Oleandrina.	Heart poison.
Opium. [Concrete juice from capsules of Papaver somniferum.] Asia, etc.	Opium. Opii Pulvis. Acet. Opii, Tinct. " Pil. " Vin. " Opii Denarcotisatum, Pulv.Ipecac et Opii, Tinct.Opii Camph., " " Deod., Ext.Op i,Emp.Opii,	Narcotina. Morphina. Codeina.	Anteperiodic and tetanic. Dose, 2 to 30 grains. Narcotic. Dose, ¼ to ½ gr. Suporific. Dose, ⅛ to ½ gr.

49

Common Name and Botanical and Geog. Source.	Officinals.	Alkaloids.	Doses and Uses.
Opium. [Concrete juice from capsules of Papaver somniferum.] Asia, etc.	Troch.Glyc.et Opii, Morphina, Morph. Acet., " Sulph., " Hydrochlor., Pulv. Morph. Co., Troch. Morph. et Ipec., Apormorphinæ Hydrochloras.	Thebaina. Narceina, and 12 other alkaloids. 'Amorphina, from Morph. + H Cl + heat.	Convulsifier and suporific. Dose, $\frac{1}{8}$ to $\frac{1}{4}$ gr. Hypnotic. Dose, $\frac{1}{2}$ to 2 grs. Emetic. Dose, $\frac{1}{60}$ to $\frac{1}{10}$ gr.
Poppy. [Papaver somniferum.] (Capsules, leaves and flowers.)		Morphia. (From capsules.)	
Pareira Brava. [Chondodendron tomentosum.] (Root.) Brazil, Peru, etc.	Pareira. Fl. Ext.	Pelosina or Cissampelina identical with Berberina.	Drug is an astringent diuretic. Dose, 30 to 60 grs.
Calabar Bean. [Physostigma venenosum.] (Seed.) W. Af.	Physostigma. Ext. and Tinct. Physostigminæ Salicylas.	Physostigmina or Éserina. Calabarina.	Arterial and nervous sedative. Dose,$\frac{1}{64}$ to $\frac{1}{12}$ gr. Tetanic. Dose, $\frac{1}{5}$ to $\frac{1}{4}$ gr.
Jaborandi. [Pilocarpus pennatifolius.] (Leaves.) So. Am.	Pilocarpus. Fl. Ext. Pilocarpinæ Hydrochloras.	Pilocarpina.	Sialogogue. Diaphoretic. Dose, $\frac{1}{8}$ to $\frac{1}{4}$ gr.
Shrubby Trefoil. [Ptelea-trifoliata.] (Bark.) N. Am.		Berberina.	Bitter tonic.
Pepper. Black Pepper. [Piper nigrum.] (Unripe fruit.) E. and W. I.	Piper. Oleores. Piperis. Piperina.	Piperina.	Antiperiodic. Dose, 1 to 8 grs.
Sabadilla. Cevadilla. [Asagræa officinalis.] (Seeds.) Mex. and So. Am.	Veratrina. Ungt. Veratrinæ.	Veratrina.	Acrid, irritant poison. Not much used internally. Dose, $\frac{1}{30}$ to $\frac{1}{12}$ grain.
Sanguinaria. Bloodroot. [Sanguinaria canadensis.] (Rhizome.) Can. and U. S.	Sanguinaria. Acet. Sang. Ext. Sang. Fl. Tinct. Sang.	Sanguinarina, like Chelerythrina from Celandine.	Stimulant, expectorant and narcotic, $\frac{1}{8}$ to $\frac{1}{4}$ gr. Dose of drug, 1 to 10 grs.

4

Common Name and Botanical and Geog. Source.	Officinals.	Alkaloids.	Doses and Uses.
Scoparius. Broom. [Sarothamnus scoparius.] (Tops.) Eu.		Sparteina. (Vol. Alk.)	Diuretic. Sedative.
Sarracenia. Pitcher-plant. Diff. var. of Sar. growing in U. S.		Sarracenina, from Sar. purpurea.	Bitter Tonic.
Sophora. [Sophora speciosa.] (Seeds.) Texas.		Sophorina.	Very poisonous. (One bean kills a man.)
Thornapple. [Datura stramonium.] (Leaves and seed.) U. S.	Stramonii Folia. " Semen. Fxt.,Fl.Ext.,Tinct.	Daturina. Like Atropia, but twice as strong.	Narcotic. Dose, $\frac{1}{120}$ to $\frac{1}{30}$ gr Leaves or root, Dose, 2 gr. Seeds, 1 gr.
Tobacco. [Nicotiana tabacum.] (Leaves.) All Temp.climates.	Tabacum.	Nicotina. (Vol. Alk.)	Narcotic, emetic, sialogogue. $\frac{1}{120}$ to $\frac{1}{30}$ grain.
Yew. [Taxus baccata.] (Leaves.) Eu.		Taxina.	Acrid poison. Dose of drug, 1 to 5 grs.
Tea. [Camellia thea.] (Leaves.) So. E., As.		Theina. Identical with Caffeina, 1.5 to 4 %.	Cerebral stimulant, sedative, etc. $\frac{1}{8}$ grain.
Theobroma. Cacao. [Theobroma cacao.] (Seeds.) Trop. Am.		Theobromina. Identical with Caffeina.	Like *last*, but stronger.
White Hellebore. [Veratrum album.] (Rhizome.) Eu.,As.,West U.S.		Jervina and Veratralbina.	Irritant poison. Dose of drug, 1 to 2 grs.
American Hellebore. Green Hellebore. [Veratrum viride.] (Rhizome.) U. S.	Veratrum Viride. Fl. Ext., Tinct.	Jervina and Veratroidina.	do.

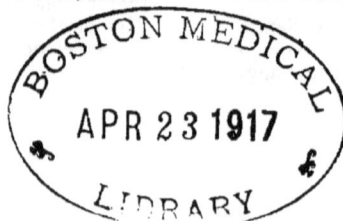

Common Name and Botanical and Geog. Source.	Officinals.	Alkaloids.	Doses and Uses.
Yellow Root. [Xanthorrhiza apiifolia.] (Rhizome and root.) U. S.		Berberina.	Bitter tonic.
Stevesacre Seed. [Delphinium staphisagria.] So. Eu.	Staphisagria.	Delphinina. .	Acrid, narcotic, poison. Dose of drug ½ grain.
Paraguay Tea. ●[Ilex paraguayensis.] (Leaves.) Brazil and Arg. Republic.		Caffeina, 1.6 %.	
Coto Bark. Source unknown. So. Am.		Vol. Alk.	

FATTY BODIES AND DERIVATIVES.

Fatty Bodies are *mostly* compound ethers, consisting of fatty acids united to the alcohol base, Glyceryl or Propenyl $C_3 H_5$. Hence they are sometimes called glycerides. Insoluble in water, sparingly soluble in alcohol, very soluble in ether, turpentine, benzole and $C S_2$. Cannot be distilled unchanged. Stearin = glyceryl + stearic acid. Margarin = do. + margaric acid. Palmitin = do. + palmitic acid. Olein = do. + oleic acid. Olein + II N O_3 = Elaidin = glyceryl + elaidic acid.

THE FOLLOWING ARE SALTS OF GLYCERYL:

Common Name.	Officinals.	Source.	Composition.
Sweet Almond Oil.	Oleum Amygdalæ Expressum. Ungt. Aquæ Rosæ. Ol. Phosphoratum.	From bitter and sweet almonds by expression. So. Eu.	Glyceryl and Oleic Acid.
Benne Oil. Gingelly Oil. Teal Oil.	Oleum Sesami.	Sesamum indicum (seeds).	Mostly Glyc. + Oleic, but contains some Palmitic & Stearic Acids.
Castor Oil.	Oleum Ricini.	Ricinus communis (seeds). U. S., etc.	Glyc. + Ricinoleic Acid.
Cod Liver Oil.	Oleum Morrhuæ.	Cod-fish, Gadus Morrhua.	Glyc. + Oleic, with some Palmitic & Stearic Acids.

Common Name.	Officinals.	Source.	Composition.
Croton Oil.	Oleum Tiglii.	Croton tiglium (seeds). So. India.	Glyc. + a number of fatty acids.
Fixed Oil of Mustard.		Sinapis alba & Sin. nigra (seeds).	Glyc. + Oleic & Erucic Acid.
Ground Nut Oil. Peanut Oil.		Arachis hypogæa. Af., S. A. & S. U. S.	Glyc. + Oleic and other acids.
Linseed Oil.	Oleum Lini.	Linum usitatissimum (seed). All temp. countries.	Glyc. + Linoleic Acid.
Bayberry Tallow. " Wax.		Myrica cerifera (berries). U. S.	Glyc. + Palmitic Acid. Fuses 116–120° F.
Cacao Butter.	Oleum Theobroma.	Theobroma Cacao (seeds). So. Am., etc.	Glyc. + Stearic and some Palmitic and Oleic Acid.
Cocoanut Oil. Oleum Cocois.		Cocos nucifera (seeds). All trop. countries.	Glyc. + Palmitic, Myristic, Lauric and other acids. Fuses at 73.4° F.
Fixed Oil of Nutmeg.		Myristica fragrans (seeds). India, etc.	Glyc. + Myristic Acid. Fuses at 113° F.
Galam Butter. Shea "		Lucuma Parkii (seeds). Cent. Af.	Glyc. + Palmitic and some Oleic Acid. Fuses at 109° F.
Illupie Oil. Indian Oil. Bassia Oil.		Bassia longifolia (seeds). India.	do.
Kokum Butter. Garcinia Oil. Mangosteen Oil.		Garcinia purpurea, etc. (seeds). Singapore.	Glyc. + Stearic, Myristic and Oleic Acid.
Lard.	Adeps. " Benzoinatus. Ceratum, Unguentum. Ceratum Resinæ, etc.	Prepared abdominal fat of Sus Scrofu.	Glyc. + Stearic and Oleic Acid. Fuses at 95° F.
Olive Oil. Sweet Oil.	Oleum Olivæ. Emp. Plumbi. Ungt. Diachylon. Cerat Camphoræ.	Olea Europea, etc. (fruit). Levant, etc.	Glyc. + Oleic, with very little Palmitic Acid.
Cotton Seed Oil.	Oleum Gossypii Seminis. Lin. Ammoniæ. Lin. Calcis. Lin. Camphoræ. Lin. Plumbi Subacet.	Gossypium herbaceum (seed). Sub-tropical climes.	Glyc. + Oleic Acid.

Common Name.	Officinals.	Source.	Composition.
Palm Oil.		Elais guineensis (fruit). W. Africa.	Glyc. + Palmitic and Oleic Acid. Fuses at 81° F.
Suet.	Sevum. Ungt. Picis Liq. " Hydrargyri.	Abdominal fat of Ovis Aries.	Glyc. + Stearic Acid. Fuses at 120° F.
Lard Oil.	Oleum Adipis. Ungt. Hyd. Nit.	From lard by expression at low temperatures.	Glyc. + Oleic Acid.

BODIES NOT CONTAINING GLYCERYL.

Common Name.	Officinals.	Source.	Composition.
Bee's Wax.	Cera Alba. Ceratum. Cerat. Cetacei. Ungt. Aq. Rosæ. Cera Flava. Ungentum. Ungt. Acid Carbol. Ungt. Hyd. Ox. Flav. Ungt. Hyd. Ox. Rub. Ungt. Mezerei. Cerat. Resinæ. " Ext. Canth. " Canth.	Honeycomb of Apis Mellifica.	Melyssyl or Myricyl + Palmitic Acid. White Wax fuses at 149° F. Yellow at 145 to 147° F.
Spermaceti.	Cetaceum. Ungt Aq. Rosæ. Cerat. Cetacei.	Sperm Whale. Physeter Macrocephalus. Pacific ocean.	Cetyl + Palmitic Acid. Fuses at 112° F.
Sperm Oil.		From the fat of do.	

DERIVATIVES.

Common Name.	Officinals.	Source.	Composition.
Oleic Acid.	Acidum Oleicum. Hydrargyri Oleatum. Veratrinæ Oleatum.	Any of the fixed oils.	

Soaps are compounds of the fatty acids with *inorganic* bases. Or, soaps are fatty bodies with glyceryl replaced by metallic bases.

Common Name.	Officinals.	Source.	Composition.
Ammonia Liniment. Hartshorn Liniment. Volatile Liniment.	Linimentum Ammoniæ.	Aq. Ammon. 30. Ol. Gossyp. Sem. 70.	Ammonia Soap.

Common Name.	Officinals.	Source.	Composition.
Castile Soap.	Sapo.	Ol. Olivæ q.s.	Soda Soap.
	Emp. Saponis.	Liq. Sodæ q.s.	Mottling due to
	Lin. Saponis.		presence of iron.
Green Soap.	Sapo Viridis.	Fixed Oil q.s.	Potash Soap.
	Tr. Saponis Viridis.	Liq. Potassa q.s.	
Lead Plaster.	Emp. Plumbi. (The	Ol. Olivæ 60.	Lead Soap.
Simple Diachylon.	base of many	Plumbi Oxidum 32.	
Litharge Plaster.	other plasters.)	Aq. q.s.	
	Ungt. Diachy-		
	lon.		
Lin.Subacet Lead.	Lin. Plumbi Suba-	Liq. Plumb. Suba-	Lead Soap.
	cetatis.	cet 40.	
		Ol. Gossyp. Sem.60.	
Lime Liniment.	Lin. Calcis.	Liq. Calcis.	Lime Soap.
Carron Oil.		Ol. Gossyp. Sem. ãã.	

GLYCERIN.

Propenyl or Glyceryl Alcohol, or Glyceryl Hydroxide, $C_3 H_5 3HO$. The sweet principle of fats. Separated in process of saponification by means of alkalies, or by super-heated steam. Sp. gr. 125. Useful as a solvent and preservative. Glycerine + $H_2 SO_4$ = Sulpho-glyceric Acid. Glycerine + HNO_3 (and $H_2 SO_4$)= Nitro-glycerin or glonoin.

Nitro-glycerin + infusorial earth, etc., = Dualin, Dynamite, etc.

Glyc. 90, Starch 10 = Glyceritum Amyli = Plasma.

" 55, Yolk of Egg 45 = " Vitelli = Glyconin.

Glycerin is used in Mucil. Trag., in many of the Extracta, Extracta Fluida, Tincturæ, etc.

GLUCOSIDAL DRUGS.

Depending wholly or in part on glucosides for their activity. Glucosides are proximate principles that yield by decomposition glucose and some other body. Some of the class are soluble in water, some in alcohol and others in ether. They are mostly harmless bitters, but some few are active poisons. *Mostly* free from N. Those containing N. are marked (N).

Common Name and Botanical and Geog. Source.	Officinals.	Glucosides.	Doses and Uses.
Apple Tree Bark. Pyrus malus. (Temp. lat.)		Phlorizin.	10 to 20 grs. Tonic.
Ash Bark. Fraximus excelsior. (Eu.)		Fraxin.	Tonic.

Common Name and Botanical and Geog. Source.	Officinals.	Glucosides.	Doses and Uses.
Aspen Bark. American Poplar. Quiver Leaf. Populus tremuloides. (No. Am.)		Populin.	Tonic. Feb.
Bearberry. Mountain Cranberry. Universe Vine. Arctostaphalos Uva-ursi. (No. Am.)	Uva Ursi. Fl. Ext.	Arbutin.	Tonic Diu. Ast. Dose, Fl. Ext., M. 20–60.
Bitter Almonds. Amygdalus communis (amara). (So. W. Eu.)	Amygdala Amara. Syrup.	Amygdalin. (N.)	17 grs. yields 50 grs. H Cy Dil.
Bittersweet. Woody Nightshade. Solanum dulcamara. (Eu.,No.Af.,As.,Am.)	Dulcamara. Fl. Ext.	Solanin. (N.) (?)	Tonic. Alt. Diu. Sud. Dose, Fl. Ext., 5ss 5j.
Black Hellebore. Helleborus niger. (Eu.)		Helleborein.	Purgative. Dose drug. 5–20 grs.
Buckthorn Bark. Eu. Buckthorn. Rhamnus Frangula. (No. Af., Eu.)	Frangula. Fl. Ext.	Frangulin.	Laxative. Dose, Fl. Ext., 5j.
Buckthorn Berries. Rhamnus catharticus. (No. As., Eu., U.S.)		Xantharhamnin.	Dose, Syr. Buckthorn Berries, 5j-5jv.
Bryony Root. Bryonia alba. " dioica. (Eu.)	Bryonia. Tinct.	Bryonin.	Hyd. Cath. Dose, drug, 10–40 grs.
Cahinca Root. Chiococca racemosa. (So. Florida and So. Am.)		Cahinchin.	Tonic, Lax., Diu. Dose, drug, 5 to to 15 grs.
Cyclamen Root. Cyclamen europeum. (So. Eu.)		Cyclamin.	Drast. purg. Dose,drug.5 grs.
Colocynth. Bitter Apple. Citrullus Colocynthis. (Cent. and W. Asia, So. Eu.)	Colocynthis. Ext., Comp. Ext.	Colocynthin.	Purgative. Dose, drug, 2–5 grs.

Common Name and Botanical and Geog. Source.	Officinals.	Glucosides.	Doses and Uses.
Elaterium. From juice of Ecbalium Elaterium. Squirting Cucumber. (So. Eu.)	Elaterinum. Trituratio Elaterini.	Elaterin.	Hyd. cath., Diu. Elaterium,$\frac{1}{8}$–$\frac{1}{4}$ gr. Elaterin,$\frac{1}{20}$–$\frac{1}{8}$gr. Trit.Elat., $\frac{1}{4}$–$\frac{1}{2}$ gr.
Foxglove. Digitalis purpurea. (Temp. lat., Eu., No. Am.)	Digitalis. Abst., Ext., Fl. Ext., Infus., Tinct.	Digitalin.	Circ. stim., Diu. Dose, leaves, 1 gr. Digitalin, $\frac{1}{80}$–$\frac{1}{30}$ gr.
Horse Chestnut. Æsculus hippocastanum. (Temp. climes.)		Æsculin.	Tonic, Feb. Dose, bark, ℥j. Æsculin, 5 grs.
Jalap. Exogonium purga. (See also resinous drugs.) (Mex.)	Jalapa. Resin, Abst., Pulv. Jalap. Co.	{ Jalapin. { Convolvulin.	Hyd.cath. Dose, drug, 10–20 grs. Resin, 3 to 6 grs.
Liquorice Root. Sweet stick. Glycyrrhiza glabra. (So.Eu., N.W. Asia.)	Glycyrrhiza. Ext.. Ext. Glyc. Purum, Fl. Ext., Pulv. Glyc Co., Glycyrrhizinum Ammon.	Glycyrrhizin.	Demul. Lax.
Monesia Bark. Chrysophyllum glycyphlœum. (So. Am.)		Glycyrrhizin and Saponin.	Stim. Ast. Dose, drug, 3 to 20 grs.
Mustard. (See React. Drugs.)		Myronic Acid.	
Mezercon Bark. (See Resin. Drugs.)		Daphnin.	
Nutgalls. Excrescences on Quercus infectorius. (So. E. Eu., etc.)	Galla. Tinct., Ungt., Acid. Tannic.	Gallo-tannin. (Tannic Acid.) Also in oak bark, etc.	Astringent. Dose, 3–10 grs.
Oak Bark (Black). Quercus tinctoria. (U. S.)		Quercitrin.	Ast.
Sarsaparilla Root. Smilax officinalis. (So. Am.)	Sarsaparilla. Dec. Sars. Co., Fl. Ext., Fl. Ext. Sars.Co., Syrup Sars. Co.	Parillin.	Alterative. Dose, drug, ℥j– ℥ij.
Senega Root. Polygala Senega. (No. Am.)	Senega. Abst.,Fl.Ext.,Syr., Syr. Scillæ Co.	Polygalic Acid (or Senegin).	Stim. Exp. Diu. Dose, root, 10– 20 g s.

Common Name and Botanical and Geog. Source.	Officinals.	Glucosides.	Doses and Uses.
Senna. Cassia acutifolia. (No. E. Af.)	Senna. Conf., Fl. Ext., Comp. Inf., Syr., Pulv. Glyc. Co., Syrup Sars. Co.	Cathartic Acid. (N.)	Cathartic. Dose, leaves, ʒss–ʒjj.
Soapwort. Bouncing Bet. Saponaria officinalis. (U. S.)		Saponin.	Alterative.
Soap Bark. Quillaia Saponaria. (So. Am.)	Quillaia.	Saponin.	Alterative.
Scammony. (See Resin. Drugs.)		Scammonin. (Same as Jalapin.)	
Trailing Arbutus. Epigœa repens. (No. Am.)		Arbutin.	Tonic, Diu. Ast. Dose, drug, ʒj.
Willow Bark. Salix alba, etc. (Temp. lat.)	Salix. Salicinum.	Salicin.	Tonic. Feb. Dose, Salicin, 10–30 grs.
Glucoside of animal origin. (From wing cases of insects.)		Chitin. (N.)	

ASTRINGENT DRUGS NOT BEFORE MENTIONED.

Depending for principal activity upon the presence of some form of tannic acid or gallic acid, but often possessing other properties.

Common Name.	Officinals.	Botanical Source and % of tannin, etc.	Geog. Source.
Agrimony.		Agrimonia eupatoria (herb). 4.75 %.	Eu., No. Am.
Alder Bark.		Alnus Serrulata. 4%.	U. S.
Alum Root.		Heuchera americana. 15 to 20 %.	No. Am.
Areca Nut. Betel-nut.		Areca Catechu (seed). 14 %.	E. I.
Bistort. Snakeweed.		Polygonum bistorta (rhizome). 21 %.	As., Eu., Am.
Blackberry.	Rubus. Ext. Rubi Fl.	Rubus villosus (bark of root).	No. Am.
Catechu. Cutch. Terra Japonica.	Catechu. Tr. Catechu Co. Trochis. Catechu.	Acacia Catechu (ext. from wood). 20 to 50 %.	E. I.

58

Common Name.	Officinals.	Botanical Source and % of tannin, etc.	Geog. Source.
Ceanothus. Red root. New Jersey tea.		Ceanothus americanus (root). 9 %.	No. Am.
Chimaphila. Prince's Pine. Wintergreen. Pipsissewa.	Chimaphila. Fl. Ext.	Chimaphila umbellata (plant). 5 %. (Also contains arbutin.)	No. Am.
Cranesbill root.	Geranium. Fl. Ext.	Geranium maculatum. 13 to 17 %.	No. Am.
Condurango.		Pseusmagenuetus equatorium (bark). 12 %.	Peru.
Galls. (See Glucosidal Drugs.)			
Gambir. Pale Catechu.		Uncaria Gambir (ext. from leaves and young shoots). 86 to 40 %.	E. I.
Hardhack. Steeple bush. Whitecap.		Spirea tomentosa (root and herb).	No. Am.
Garcinia. Mangosteen.		Garcinia mangostana, etc. (bark and fruit rind).	E. I.
Kino.	Kino. Tr. Kino.	Pterocarpus Marsupium. (Inspissated juice from incisions in trunk.)	India.
Logwood.	Hæmatoxylon. Ext. Hæmatoxyli.	Hæmatoxylon campechianum (heart wood).	Cent. Am. and W. I.
Myrobalans.		Terminalia chebula (fruit). 40 %.	India.
Oak Bark.	Quercus Alba.	Quercus alba (bark).	Temp. lat.
Persimmons.		Diospyros virginiana (unripe fruit).	U. S.
Pomegranate Rind.		Punica Granatum (rind of fruit). 28%.	So. W. Asia.
Pomegranate Bark.	Granatum.	Punica Granatum (bark of root). 22 %.	So. W. Asia.
Rhatany.	Krameria. Ext., Fl.Ext.,Tinct.	Krameria triandria. Krameria tomentosa.	Peru.
Pale Rose Leaves.	Rosa Centifolia. Aq,, Syr. Sars. Co.	Rosa centifolia (petals).	W. Asia, etc.
Red Rose Leaves.	Rosa Gallica. Conf., Fl.Ext., Syr., Mel., Pil. Aloës et Myrrh.	Rosa Gallica (petals).	So. Eu., etc.

59

Common Name.	Officinals.	Botanical Source and % of tannin, etc.	Geog. Source.
Sumach.	Rhus Glabra. Ext. Rhois Glabræ Fl.	Rhus glabra (berries).	No. Am.
Sweet Fern. Fern Gale.		Comptonia asplenifolia (leaves and tops). 8 %.	Can. & U. S.
Witch Hazel.	Hamamelis. Ext. Hamamelidis Fl.	Hamamelis virginica (leaves). 8 %.	Can. & U. S.

UNCLASSED DRUGS.

Common Name and Geog. Source.	Officinals.	Botanical Source.	Activity.
Alder Bark. Black Alder. (U. S.)	Prinos.	Prinos verticillatus.	Bitter prin. and ast. Tonic and ast. Dose, 30 to 60 grs.
Aloes. (E. Af. and W. Arabia.)	Aloe. Aloe Purif. Ext. Aloës Aquosum.	Aloe Socotrina. (Inspissated juice of leaves).	Bitter prin., a resin (?). (Socaloin.) Cathartic. Dose, 2-10 grs.
Purified Aloes.	Aloe Purificata. Pil. Al., Pil. Al. et Asaf., Pil. Al. et Ferri, Pil. Al. et Mast., Pil. Al. et Myrrh, Tr. Aloës, Tr. Al. et Myrrh, Vin Aloës, Tr. Benz. Co.	From Aloe.	
Azedarach. (North India. Cult. So. U. S.)	Azedarach.	Melia Azedarach (bark of root).	Bitter resin (?). " alkaloid (?). Cath., Emet., Anthel.
Black Haw. (U. S.)	. Viburnum. Fl. Ext.	Viburnum prunifolium (bark).	Bitter resin (?). Tannic Acid. Ton. Antispas. Nerv. Dose, Fl. Ext. 3j-3ij.
Blue Flag. (U. S.)	Iris. Ext., Fl. Ext.	Iris versicolor (rhizome and rootlets).	Resin. Alkaloid (?). Cath. Emet., Alt., Diu. Dose, 10 to 20 grs. Dose, Irisin, the resinoid or oleoresin, 3 to 4 grs.

Common Name and Geog. Source.	Officinals.	Botanical Source.	Activity.
Butternut. (U. S.)	Juglans. Ext.	Juglans cinerea (inner bark of root).	Bitter Extrative, etc. Cathertic, Alt. Dose, Ex., 5 to 20 grs.
Cassia Fistula. Purging Cassia. (Trop. countries. India,W. I., etc.)	Cassia Fistula. Conf Semæ.	Cassia Fistula (fruit).	Laxative. Dose, ʒij +.
Chestnut Leaves. (Eu. and No. Am.)	Castanea. Fl. Ext.	Castanea vesca (leaves).	(?). Used for whooping cough. Dose, Fl. Ext. 20 to 60 m.
Chiretta. Chirata. (No. Ind.)	Chirata. F. Ext., Tr.	Ophelia Chirata (entire plant).	Neut. bitter prin. Chiratin. A bitter acid— ophelic. Tonic. Dose, Fl. Ext., 20 to 60 m.
Corn Smut. (Temp. climes.)	Ustilago.	Ustilago Maydis (fungi grown upon Zea Mays).	Sclerotic acid (?). Alkaloid (?). Abortifacient. Dose, 10–60 grs.
Couch-grass. Quick-grass. (Eu., U. S.)	Triticum. Fl. Ext.	Triticum repens (rhizome).	(?). Diuretic. Dose, Fl. Ext., ʒj +.
Dandelion. (Temp. climes, etc.)	Taraxacum. Ext., Fl. Ext.	Taraxacum Densleonis (root).	Bitter neut. prin. Taraxacin. Tonic, Diu., Aper. Dose, drug, ʒj +.
Dogwood. (U. S.)	Cornus. Fl. Ext.	Cornus Florida (bark of root).	Bitter neut. prin. Cornin. Tonic and ast. Dose, Fl.Ext.20–60m.
Ergot. (Temp. climes.)	Ergota. Ext., Fl. Ext., Vin.	The sclerotium of the fungus Clavicips purpurea, replacing the grain of Secale cereale.	Sclerotic Acid, Ergotinine (?), Scleromucin, Ecboline. Abortifacient, etc. Dose, ʒss–ʒij.
Fig. (So. Eu.)	Ficus. Conf. Sennæ	Fleshy receptacle of Ficus Carica.	Sugar and gum.
Gentian. (Eu.)	Gentiana. Ext., Fl. Ext. Tr. Gent. Co.	Gentiana lutea (root).	Bitter principle. Gentio-picrin. Tonic. Dose, Fl. Ext.30–60 m.

Common Name and Geog. Source.	Officinals.	Botanical Source.	Activity.
Goa Powder. Araroba. (Brazil, So. Am,)	Chrysarobinum, a mixture of proximate principles, commonly known as chrysophanic acid. Ungt. Chrysarobini.	Goa powder is a substance found deposited in the wood of the trunk of Andria Araroba.	Purgative. Dose, 5–25 grs. Used externally, in skin disorders.
Gutta-Percha. (E. I.)	Gutta-Percha. Liq.Gutta-Perchæ.	Concrete exudation of Isonandra Gutta.	Externally.
Lactucarium. (Eu.)	Lactucarium. Fl. Ext., Syr.	Concrete milk juice of Lactuca virosa.	Bitter prin., lactucic acid, etc. Soporific. Dose, Fl. Ext. 5–30 m.
Male Fern. (Eu., As., No. Af., W. U. S.)	Aspidium. Oleores. Aspidii.	Aspidium Felixmas. Aspidium marginale (rhizome).	Oleoresin. Remedy for tape worm. Dose, Oleores,$\bar{3}$ss-$\bar{3}$j.
Pansy. Violet.	Viola Tricolor.	Viola tricolor (flowering herb).	Laxative.
Pumpkin Seed.	Pepo.	Cucurbita Pepo (seed).	Resin. For tape worm. Dose, $\bar{3}$jss of seeds.
Poke Berry. Garget.	Phytplaccæ Bacca.	Phytolacca decandra.	Emet., Purg., Narc. (?).
Poke Root. Garget.	Phytolaccæ Radix.	Phytolacca decandra.	Emet., Purg., Nar. (?). Dose, 1–5 grs.
Picrotoxin.	Picrotoxinum.	Neut. prin., from seeds of Anamirta paniculata. (India.) (Cocculus Indicus. Fish berries.)	Acrid narcot. Dose, $\frac{1}{60}$–$\frac{1}{8}$ gr.
Poison Oak. (No. Am.)	Rhus Toxicodendron.	Rhus Toxicodendron (fresh leaves).	Toxicodendric Acid. Stim. narcot.
Pulsatilla. (Eu., Temp. climes.)	Pulsatilla.	Anemone Pulsatilla. Anemone pratensis (herb).	Acrid neut. prin. Anemonin. Emmenagogue, etc. Dose, drug, 2–3 grs.
Quassia. Bitter Ash. (W. I.)	Quassia. Ext., Fl. Ext., Tr.	Picræna excelsa (wood).	Bitter neut. prin. Quassin. Tonic, Dose, Fl. Ext., 5–10 m.

Common Name and Geog. Source.	Officinals.	Botanical Source.	Activity.
Queen's Root. Stillingia. (U. S.)	Stillingia. Fl. Ext.	Stillingia sylvatica (root).	Vol. oil, etc. (?). Alt., Emet., Cath. Dose, powder, 15–30 grs.
Rhubarb. (Ind., China, etc.)	Rheum. Ext., Fl. Ext., Pil., Syr., Tinct.,Vin., Pil. Rhei Co., Pulv. Rhei Co., Syr. Rhei Aro., Tr. Rhei Aro., Tr. Rhei Dulc.	Rheum officinale, etc.	Resinous prin. Phæoretin and Erythroretin. Also, Emodin and Chrysophanic acid, etc. Cath. and Ast. Dose, 5 to 15 grs.
Raspberry. (Temp. climes.)	Rubus Idæus. Syr.	Rubus idæus (fruit).	Acid flavor.
Red Saunders. (India.)	Santalum Rubrum. Tr. Lav. Co.	Pterocarpus santalinus (wood).	Res. col. matter. Santalin. For color.
Squill. (So. Eu.)	Scilla. Acet., Syr., Fl. Ext., Tr., Syr. Scil. Co.	Urginea Scilla (sliced bulb).	Bit. prin, scillitin, oil, etc. (?). Expec., Diu., Emet. Dose, 1–3 grs.
Thoroughwort. Boneset. (U. S.)	Eupatorium.	Eupatorium perfoliatum (leaves and flowering tops).	Bitter prin. Tonic Diaph. Dose, 20–30 grs
Wahoo. Burning bush. (U. S.)	Euonymus. Ext.	Euonymus atropurpureus (bark).	Bitter prin. Euonymin, Laxative, etc. Dose, ℨss–ℨj.
Yellow Dock.	Rumex. Fl. Ext.	Rumex crispus, etc. (root).	(?). Tonic, Alt., Ast. Dose, Fl. Ext., ℨss–ℨj.
Vanilla. (W. I., Mex., S. A.)	Vanilla. Tr., Trochis. Ferri.	Vanilla planifolia (fruit).	Bitter extractive, vanillin, etc. Flavor, stim.

ANIMAL DRUGS NOT BEFORE MENTIONED.

Common Name.	Officinals.	Source and Use.
Ambergris. (Ambra Grisea).		A morbid product of the sperm whale—Physeter macrocephalus. Antispasmodic. Dose, 5–10 grs.

Common Name.	Officinals.	Source and Use.
Cantharis.	Cantharis.	Cantharis vesicatoria.
Spanish Flies.	Cerat., Cerat. Ext. Canth., Charta Canth., Collod. cum Canth., Lin. Canth., Emp. Picis cum Canth., Tinct.	*Internally*, powerful stimulant to urinary and genital organs in small doses. In large, irritant poison. *Externally*, vesicant. Activity— cantharidin, a neut. prin., white and cryst.
Castor.		Beaver—Castor fibre. (Dried preputial follicles and secretion.) Nerv. stim. Dose, 10 grains.
Cochineal.	Coccus.	Dried female of Coccus Cacti. (Color.)
Egg Albumen. (Albumen Ovi.)	Test Solution of Albumen.	White of egg of Gallus Bankiva, var domesticus.
Egg Yolk.	Vetellus. Glyceritum Vitelli Mist. Chlorof.	Yolk of egg, do.
Gelatin. Gelatina. Glutin.		From bone cartilage, hide trimmings, tendons, etc. Best sort = gelatin. Poorer sort = glue. Used for court plaster, capsules, pill coating, etc., etc.
Isinglass. Fish-glue.	Ichthyocolla. Emp.Ichthyocollæ. Test Sol. Gelatin.	Swimming bladders of sturgeons. Acipenser Hugo.
Milk. (Lac.)		From cow,—Bos Taurus. Nutrient, etc.
Musk.	Moschus. Tinct. Moschi.	Musk deer,—Moschus moschiferus. Dried secretion of preputial follicles. Nerv. stim. and antispas. Dose, 10 grs.
Ox gall. Beef bile.	Fel Bovis. Fel Bovis Inspissatum. Fel Bovis Purificatum.	Gall of ox—Bos Taurus. Tonic and laxative. Dose, 5 to 10 grs.
Pepsin.	Pepsinum Saccharatum. Liquor Pepsini.	Digestive principle of gastric juice, obtained from mucous membrane of the stomach of the hog (etc.). Digestive. Dose, 5 to 30 grs.
Pancreatin.		From pancreatic juice (pancreas of Bos Taurus).
Rennet.		*Usually* fourth stomach of calf (Bos Taurus), salted, dried, etc.

www.ingramcontent.com/pod-product-compliance
Lightning Source LLC
Chambersburg PA
CBHW021826190326
41518CB00007B/754